PANDEMIC

EFFECTS ON LATIN AMERICA AND THE INTERACTIONS WITH CHINA

Carlos Aquino
Ignacio Bartesaghi/ Natalia De Maria
Oscar Olvido Cabrera
Lucas Vitor de Carvalho Sousa/ Silvina Regina de Souza Rojas
Marcos Cordeiro/ Luis Antonio Paulino
Nicole Jordan Prudencio
Wilson Lopez-López
Jorge Malena
Pedro Monzon Barata
Milton Reyes Herrera
Ricardo Santana Friedli
Eduardo Tzili-Apango
Jose Luis Valenzuela

Fernando Reyes Matta (Editor)

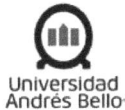

Universidad
Andrés Bello.

PANDEMIC:
EFFECTS ON LATIN AMERICA AND THE
INTERACTIONS WITH CHINA

First Edition: September 2020

© Fernando Reyes Matta
© Centro de Estudios Latinoamericanos sobre China
   Universidad Andrés Bello

ISBN: 978-1-953903-00-6

Editor: Fernando Reyes Matta

© of this Edition:
Fernando Reyes Matta
Long Publishing
www.ai60.com

First Printing November 2020/Printed in the United States of America

http://internacional.unab.cl/direccion-de-relaciones-internacionales/celc/

CONTENTS

II

Milton Reyes Herrera

Presentation

The Covid-19 pandemic is a phenomenon that has hit all countries and has also become a challenge for the continuity of our tasks in every sphere of life. Along with adapting the educational curricula to online teaching, we have also been called on to study, as we implement this modality, its ongoing effects on Uruguay, other Latin American countries, and the rest of the world. This is because, in line with the development strategy of Andres Bello University, we understand internationalization as the incorporation of a global, intercultural and international component in all of the University's goals. Thus it was with special interest that we welcomed the opportunity to carry out a joint analysis with other Latin American universities of the impact of this pandemic, the social and economic effects that it has ushered in, including as a study variable the ties with China in the sphere of health and other areas of cooperation born of this circumstance.

This book, sponsored and published by our University's Center of Latin American Studies on China, is the fruit of that joint work. Fourteen universities of Mexico, Central America (El Salvador), Cuba, Colombia, Brazil, Argentina, Uruguay, Peru, Bolivia, Ecuador, and our University in Chile undertook an academic effort to grasp, from the perspective of our immediate environment, an interpretation of the changes that the pandemic has generated, the realities it has brought to light, the health programs implemented, and the challenges that the events have brought to bear on the application of emergency programs within the different realities of the region. Reading these works shows us the gamut of reactions from the different countries, ranging from denial of what loomed ahead, to the rapid, efficient execution of programs.

From the Department of International Relations of Andres Bello University, we consider this work an important contribution to the idea of a Latin America summoned to work more unitedly, in a more coordinated way, because the challenges signified by a world in the midst of deep change are calling us to the task. We are aware that at this moment in time many rifts are evident in Latin America, and the region is in urgent need of rearticulating itself as a whole, if we wish to be a part of reorganizing the international order. We are likewise aware of how bipolarity has emerged on the international scene, and thus our task is to train professionals capable of grasping all the realities that await their engagement and sound action. Inspired by this goal, we encourage our departments to strengthen their ties beyond our borders and promote international research, build bonds through developing joint projects with other universities abroad, promoting the mobility of our academics and the permanent search for new agreements that can add value to the training of our students.

Just as it behooves us to understand the evolution of the western world and our continent, we have also taken on the challenge of understanding the unfolding of other realities, such as that of China. The importance that this Asian power has acquired for humanity's contemporary development is undeniable. Chile is well aware of this, as China has become our primary business partner, followed by the U.S. and the European Union. All of these developments as a whole call for us to adopt a very pluralistic gaze, and we are working toward establishing agreements with the best universities of China. This book is the result of a dialog, and the prestige gained by our Center, which is dedicated to China, has enabled its Director, Fernando Reyes Matta, to meet with a ready response from renowned academics, who agreed to participate in this collective publication. We thank them for their contributions, which strengthen our University's goal of growing internationalization.

Fabiola Novoa Caamaño
Director
Office of International Relations
Universidad Andrés Bello

I. Introduction
Latin America-China: A Changed Perception of Distance

Fernando Reyes Matta[1]

Some might say that this book has been written without a complete and pertinent perspective, after more time was allowed to pass for observing the events' unfolding and their outcomes. However, upon reading each guest scholar's work, it is clear that writing amid the unfolding events gives their words emotionality, richness and the informational immediacy of a critical moment for Latin America. A moment in which the pandemic arrived, following its appearance in China, crossed the Middle East and Europe, and finally traversed the Atlantic with the first case detected in Sao Paulo, Brazil. Starting in March, its impact became especially critical and the Latin American countries initiated the application of diverse policies, which ranged from Brazil's denial, to rigorous quarantines in Argentina, Chile and other countries of the region.

By then China had already brought the pandemic's expansion throughout its territory under control and was in a position to offer support to other countries, thanks to the experience gained by her doctors, health personnel, architects and engineers. She

1. Director of the Center for Latin American Studies on China (Centro de Estudios Latinoamericanos sobre China, CELC), Universidad Andrés Bello, Chile.

was also able to disclose the effects on the economy of the strict measures adopted in response to the health crisis. At the same time, the reactions of the U.S. government, in tense discussions with scientists and specialists in epidemics such as Covid-19 were being followed with some disconcertment on our continent. More than once President Donald Trump's declarations seemed to border on delirium while his words found echo only in President Jair Bolsonaro, who, despite repeated evidence to the contrary, continued to meet with Trump supporters and consort with them. However, the numbers were convincing. As of July 20, the U.S. had recorded 145,000 deaths and Brazil, 81,500, and their numbers of infected were also the highest in the world—4,026,000 in the U.S. and 2,167,000 in Brazil.

From the perspective of the Latin American countries, the 2020 pandemic showed a U.S. in absentia, removed from the cooperation programs of the past, versus a China that was present through various forms of engagement and cooperation. The Asian country became their primary supplier of equipment, masks, sanitary clothing and other supplies. China also made her proximity felt through various video-conferences and webinars, during which Chinese doctors initiated a direct dialog with Latin American doctors and public health experts. In the course of these past months, China's relations with Latin America have demonstrated that physical distance is no longer a major obstacle; the rationales and opportunities for contact around shared issues in a common agenda have effectively cancelled it. One example: the events organized within the framework of the relationship between CELAC and China. A videoconference was held on March 24 (the evening of the 23rd of March in Latin America), attended by representatives of 25 countries and their Chinese counterparts, who were led by the Vice President of China's National Health Commission, Zeng Yixin.

CELAC-China: Let's Watch What Happens

A special meeting on Covid-19 was organized by the foreign affairs ministers of China and of Mexico, Wang Yi and Marcelo Ebrard, the latter in his capacity as the head of Mexico's international relations and coordinator of CELAC this year. At the zoom meeting, the participating foreign ministers and/or their representatives attended a special session of the CELAC-China Forum, to report on how their countries were responding to the pandemic, and shared their respective visions of the region's economic reality and its linkages with the global economy. Trade tensions are among the region's concerns, the changes in trade flows for the countries that are exporters of raw materials, as well as the obstacles in the service areas, especially in tourism, a major income source for the Caribbean countries.[2]

2. https://www.infobae.com/américa/mexico/2020/07/23/china-prestara-usd-1000-millones-a- mexico-américa-latina-y-el-caribe-para-la-compra-de-vacunas-contra-el-covid-19/

Aside from Ministers Ebrard and Wang Yi, also present at the digital meeting were high-ranking representatives of Argentina, Barbados, Chile, Colombia, Costa Rica, Cuba, Dominican Republic, Ecuador, Panama, Peru, Trinidad and Tobago, and Uruguay.

Minister Ebrard also thanked the Chinese government and its partners in Latin America and the Caribbean for supporting the resolution submitted to the U.N. General Assembly on international cooperation to ensure global access to medicines, vaccines and medical equipment for the response to COVID-19. The resolution was adopted by the U.N. with the co-sponsorship of 179 countries. The minister also expressed his conviction that the priority for the next few months needed to be actions to develop treatments and vaccines, aside from creating effective mechanisms for their universal distribution.

"The resolution was an important expression of solidarity and political commitment that we must now transform into action," said Minister Ebrard to his peers.

For his part, Minister Wang Yi, who is also a member of the Chinese Council of State, expressed thanks for the cooperation of the Latin American countries during the most difficult time of the pandemic in China. He later pointed out that China was ready to work with Latin America to face the multiple challenges posed by COVID-19, and to make a shared contribution to global economic recovery. The political concept implicit in the words "shared contribution" is no small matter, as the idea spreads around the world that we have entered a stage of international reorganization in multiple spheres. Minister Wang indicated that since the start of the epidemic, China and Latin America have overcome the obstacle of distance and have undertaken actions of integrated cooperation in the fight against the virus. The high-ranking Chinese official additionally emphasized, as was announced in Ecuador, Mexico and other countries in the region, that the vaccine currently being developed in China would be "a universally accessible public good, and credits totaling US$1 billion will be allocated to facilitate access to it of the region's nations". From Beijing it was communicated that the ministers also expressed "their opposition to politicizing or stigmatizing the epidemic, and their willingness to work with China to deepen cooperation in all fields, and promote integral partnerships of cooperation between Latin America and China to elevate cooperation to a new level."[3] In mid-April, the official international broadcaster of the U.S. government, the Voice of America, reported on a meeting held by the Council of the Americas, a business institution that is highly influential in hemispheric relations, on the current situation in the region. The institution's analysis referred to the presence of China in the region and its ramifications. "As Vice President of the Council of the Americas Eric Farnsworth has emphasized, this entire

3. http://mx.china-embassy.org/esp/xw/t1800569.html

scenario has placed China in a position in which, in comparison to how other countries formulate policy, she seeks to demonstrate that she can move her goals and ideals forward, as shown with the reopening of Wuhan," the report stated. In the introduction to the analysis, the following question was formulated: "Quite apart from the working classes and the internal economies of the affected countries, the powers of the world are reinventing themselves and likewise seeking positions of power. How will the relationship between China and the Latin American Region move forward?"[4]

A good portion of the information that has circulated through Latin America in the first months of 2020, in referring to China, has described the Asian country as a purveyor. It was no easy matter to gain access to all the resources that China was producing almost in exclusivity; the countries did not formulate a common policy in this respect, neither the European countries, nor those of Latin America. Each country sought to carry out operations under cover of secrecy to prevent the requisitioning of consignments before they reached their final destination, as happened in France and in the U.S. However, there can be no doubt that the process of interaction between "Pandemic-Latin American reality - China" constitutes a field of analysis that requires more substantial and diverse contributions. Clearly,

4. https://www.voanoticias.com/américa-latina/eeuu-china-latinoamérica-comercio-covid-corona- virus

for the Latin American countries, cultivating ties with China is an increasingly nuanced challenge of maintaining political and diplomatic balance against the backdrop of growing tensions between the U.S. and the Asian power.

The links between China and her counterparts on the continent have been progressively reinforced by declarations or defining moments, with more wide-reaching and subtle significations than is apparent at a surface level. One instance of this is the joint declaration issued by Chile's Ministry of Foreign Affairs and China's Ministry of Trade on July 17, aimed at mitigating the effects of Covid-19 on international commerce and investment, accelerating the reestablishment of the common economic and trade order, and promoting the long-term development of international trade and investment. The two countries called for close, coordinated cooperation to face the pandemic, "with a firm commitment to presenting a united front before Covid-19 in matters of the economy and trade, and to oppose trade protectionism". In other words, the effectiveness of the Free Trade Agreement between the two countries that was recently raised to a higher level served as the frame of reference for the pandemic's challenges to future developments on the economic front. Here are the report's main paragraphs:

"The two countries recognize the importance of trade and investment liberalization at this critical time, keeping global supply chains open and connected. Both countries will work to guarantee the free flow of trade and ensure that foreign trade lines and critical infrastructure remain open, including the use of air and sea transport routes. The two countries recognize the importance of the Free Trade Agreement (FTA) for promoting the growth of bilateral trade and investment and the sustained development of both countries. Since the two parties' signing of the TLC in 2005 and the Protocol in 2017, we have witnessed the rapid growth of trade and investment in both countries. Our trade grew from US$ 7 billion in 2005, the year of the signing, to US$41 billion in 2019 (480% growth). Both parties will closely collaborate to better implement our bilateral FTA, which plays an important role in facilitating the free flow of goods and services, to support the integrity of global supply chains, mitigate the impacts of the pandemic on bilateral trade and investment, and contribute to more sustainable post-crisis economic growth. The two countries will adopt the necessary measures to ensure the continuous flow of vital medical supplies and equipment, critical agricultural products and other cross-border goods and services required to protect the health of our citizens. They will work together to assist vulnerable developing countries and less-developed countries. Both countries make a commitment to supporting the Multilateral Trade System and agree that the emergency measures for tackling COVID-19 must be concrete, transparent and temporary, and should also be compatible with the rules established by the WTO."[5]

If Chile is an important business partner (not so much in terms of volume but of the areas of products it supplies to China-especially copper, fruit, wood and forestry products), Mexico is another important country for the development of China's presence in Latin America, particularly this year. The trade dialog has always been difficult because of the strong imbalance in China's favor, and, of course, the fact that 85% of Mexico's trade is with the U.S. However, the Mexican government has always maintained an interest in seeking some type of strategic relationship with China, an interest that China shares. Given that in 2020 Mexico took on the role of president pro tempore of CELAC, which, notwithstanding a decline in recent years, still maintains a special Forum with China, the government of President López Obrador has set itself the goal of strengthening these ties while at the same time managing the rapprochement with Washington after signing the new Free Trade Agreement or T-MEC. The T-MEC additionally links Mexico to Canada. Opportunities for outreach have arisen thanks to Covid-19, not just for bilateral assistance, but also for planning diplomatic and expert meetings of the CELAC-China Forum.

5. https://www.subrei.gob.cl/2020/07/declaracion-conjunta-para-fortalecer-la-cooperacion-en-el- marco-del-tlc-y-combatir-el-covid-19-entre-el-ministerio-de-comercio-de-china-y-el-ministe- rio-de-relaciones-exteriores-de-chile/

Air Bridges and Multiple Webinars: Something Changed

Against this backdrop it is worth noting two developments in China's relations with the Latin American countries, since the intensification of the pandemic's impact on this region: (a) the creation of various air bridges from South America and Mexico; (b) the utilization of digital platforms such as Zoom to organize multiple meetings in a novel format.

The air bridge between China and Mexico to provide supplies to Mexican hospitals during the COVID-19 pandemic is considered by both governments a milestone in their cooperative relations. On June 28 an initial phase was completed of 21 flights, and a second one was immediately scheduled for 20 more. For two-and-a-half months, cargo planes flew into Mexico City from Shanghai. The first 20 flights landed with tens of tons of material that Mexico acquired from Chinese companies, while the second stage of the air bridge began with a special consignment of supplies donated by China to the Mexican people. "A significant symbolic act that establishes a new milestone of cooperation in the difficult times we are living through," said Marta Delgado, Mexican Undersecretary of Multilateral Affairs, from the capital city's airport upon the completion of the plan, praising "the 21 flights of the air bridge between Mexico and Shanghai". For his part, Chinese

Ambassador Zhu Qingqiao pointed out that COVID-19 does not respect borders and all are part of a community with a shared future-a central concept of China's foreign policy. Thus, union and cooperation are required to deal with the pandemic and achieve economic recovery. "China and Mexico will promote bilateral cooperation while emphasizing equality and mutual benefit," Ambassador Zhu said, adding, "the Chinese side will reinforce communications with actions such as the resumption of productive activities and economic reactivation."

In Mexico, the route between the Mexican capital and Shanghai is already an established one of Aero Mexico's flights. But the situation was different for Aerolíneas Argentinas and LATAM flights, as these airlines had never before flown directly to China. The China Plan was started up with the experience christened as "the Solidarity Jet". LATAM landed in the airports of Shanghai, Beijing, Guangdong and Fujian, a total of 24 flights broken down into 13 round trips from and to Chile (not all of them charters). The same number of flights lifted off from Brazil and there were two flights to Peru in an inter-airline modality for transporting masks, fast tests for COVID-19 and medicines. Additionally, there were three flights that flew from South Korea to Colombia. Two Boeing jets, a 787 and a 777, were retrofitted, removing the seats for more cargo capacity in the cabin. More than 30 persons carried out each cargo mission. Flight durations averaged 60 to 70 hours in all, depending on whether the final destination was Chile or Brazil.

LATAM's website explains that a complex procedure had to be put in place for the air bridge to coordinate logistics, from obtaining the required flight permits from governments—which in normal times can take months—to landing in the airports, refueling and coordinating cabin crews and ground support crews. Additionally, the number of seats on each flight was limited and thus priority had to be assigned to pilots and ground operators who had to perform support tasks aboard each aircraft. When in China, the airline company also outsourced the work of the ground support teams, which then posed the challenge of the language barrier and differences in work procedures. This all needed to be done while racing against time, since the volume of flight traffic and cargo operations allowed each aircraft no more than five hours' parking on the tarmac.[6]

The air bridge was a completely new experience for Aerolíneas Argentinas (AA). The airline's customary route was to fly to Sydney, Australia, skirting the Polar Circle. The air bridge meant that AA had to fly farther north along a corridor similar to one used by LATAM flights. On April 18, the first flight of what was termed a historical "air bridge" landed at Ezeiza International Airport in Buenos Aires, arriving from the Chinese city of Shanghai with a donation from China of

6. https://asialink.américaeconomia.com/sociedad/latam-realiza-puente-aereo-por-covid-19-en- tre-latinoamérica-y-china

13 tons of supplies, such as medical and personal protection material against COVID-19. The operation was described by the authorities as "yet another demonstration of the friendship and cooperation that exists between both countries".

To carry out the initiative, Airbus 330-200 jets had to be especially adapted, equipped with container nets to transport 84% more cargo than a normal passenger flight. "This is a very emotional situation for us and we're extremely content, satisfied and deeply moved. We all know nowadays how complicated it is to obtain equipment and personal protection items in the midst of this pandemic," said Axel Kicillof, Governor of the Province of Buenos Aires, as he welcomed the first returning flight.

The captain of the Argentine aircraft as well as the Chileans on board all said that it was their first direct flight to and from China. The AA flights' total duration was 56 hours with a stopover for refueling in Auckland, Australia. The flight crews were made up of 12 pilots and co-pilots, four technicians and two dispatchers in charge of coordinating the cargo operations. On each flight the crew remained aboard the aircraft, which was allowed to park on the runway for just five hours, load its cargo and fly back.

An open-ended question has emerged regarding a possible future plan for after the airlift, namely, whether it will be possible to establish regular direct commercial flights in future between Santiago or Buenos Aires and Shanghai. The question is open-ended, born of the precedent of these flights in response to the pandemic-an experience that has sown seeds for a possible future.

The other reality that has been the stimulus for unusual experiences is the use of digital networks and the Cloud.

Never before these recent months of 2020 have there been so many conferences and direct dialogs held between Latin America and China.

We have already mentioned the medical conferences and the ministerial meeting of the CELAC-China Forum.

However, there have been many more such instances and it is possible to assert that because of the coronavirus, China opened up the Digital Route of its relationship with the Latin American countries.

At this time, the Internet communications between China and Latin America and the Caribbean are happening at different levels and between different actors, for varied purposes.

The clearest form of digital communication available today on both sides of the globe are webinars or web conferencing, for online interaction between participants through applications installed on mobile devices or computers.

Language barriers have been sorted out through simultaneous translation or the use of English.

Time differences have been accommodated by assuming that 9:00 a.m. is 9:00 p.m. in another country and within this framework the appropriate coordinations are carried out. An example of these interactions was the conference held with Chief Engineer Yu Di Hua of General Contracting Company, a subsidiary of Grupo China Construction Third Engineering Bureau Co. Ltd. (CCTEB). The engineer "was head of the design management and technical administration of the Huo Shen Shan Hospital, a field hospital complex built in just 10 days as a clinical response to COVID-19 patients in Wuhan, China".

All of those interested in learning more about this exceptional construction received explanations, images and direct responses from a major protagonist in the project.

The meeting was organized by the Technology Development Corporation of the Chilean Chamber of Construction (*Cámara Chilena de la Construcción,* CChC) and the Chinese Council for the Promotion of International Trade of Hubei Province (CCPIT - HUBEI).

The meeting was attended by over 150 construction experts.

Universities have also moved on to a different stage of relations through this medium.

And by the way, not just with China.

However, at the center of the interactions between the Asian country and the Latin American academic centers, novel elements have unfolded.

For example, the dialog held by Tsinghua University with three ambassadors-of Argentina, Brazil and Chile-on their views regarding the current gaze directed at China, the ways of dealing with Covid-19, and China's perspectives on the international stage.

It was organized by Taotao Chen, Director of the Center Latin America Tsinghua University. The interviewees were Marcos Caramuru de Paiva of Brazil, Diego Ramirez Guelar from Argentina, and the author, who participated in representation of Chile.

The interesting thing is that the interviews were seen by an audience that was a significant contingent of students from different countries taking part via Zoom, who were also attending the Tsinghua University Summer Program.

In China, this already widely-accepted new form of dialog is called "communication on the Cloud".

Pueblo Online included the following special news announcement:

"Against the special backdrop of the epidemic, President Xi Jinping, as the country's guide and the people's leader, has maintained close contact and communication with the leaders of many Latin American countries, including Brazil, Argentina, Cuba, Mexico, Chile and Venezuela, which has consolidated the fundamental cornerstone for developing the relations between China and Latin America in this new situation, lighting the way towards our relationships in the future".

In addition to the regional fora organized with the

participation of Minister Wang Yi, smooth bilateral exchanges have taken place through the Internet. Events such as the 17th Meeting of Policy Consultations between the Ministries of Foreign Affairs of China and Mexico, the 3rd Meeting of the Permanent Intergovernmental Commission between China and Argentina, and the 2nd Meeting of Policy Consultations between the Ministries of Foreign Affairs of China and Panama were successfully held in virtual format.

Both experiences—the air bridges and the digital video conferences—are the cornerstones of a new mode of interaction between China and the countries of Latin America. The path forward has been left open for future such meetings between diverse institutions of civil society, provincial bodies, or between political parties. With the epidemic's spread across Latin America, China has actively coordinated communications between its provinces and cities with over 10 Latin American countries, including Argentina, Chile, Panama, Costa Rica, El Salvador, holding "one-on-one" video-conferences with experts. In response to the pandemic, China has held special meetings with undersecretaries of foreign affairs from the Caribbean countries that maintain diplomatic relations with China, and organized virtual meetings with the Latin American countries to exchange experiences in epidemic control and prevention.

The 127th Canton Fair has transitioned from its classic modality, which has been phased out, to holding the event on the cloud and attracting a large number of visitors from Latin America. The Chinese companies have developed live broadcast plans for the time zones of the Latin American continent and are holding integrated showroom exhibits of their products. Latin American buyers can now conduct business without leaving home.

A Chinese company that markets medical devices and that participated in the fair for the first time received an order for US$ 80,000 from Ecuador just ten minutes after the live broadcast.

The China Council for the Promotion of International Trade held the China-Latin America (Mexico) International Digital Trade Fair, inviting over 2,000 Chinese companies and over 5,000 Latin American buyers to the Fair. Macrodata was used to facilitate accurate matching and offer online negotiation services. The event achieved a total commercial volume of US$8.02 million.

With this scenario of transformations and actions deployed at the same time as the events were occurring, the possibility arose for the Universidad Andrés Bello Center of Latin American Studies on China to invite academics from various countries of the region to share their reflections with us, enriched with the data at hand on the impact of the pandemic on their milieux.

It was imperative to consider the economic and social trends already unfolding before the advent of Covid-19, the inequalities that had generated social protests in countries such as Chile and Colombia; but, above all, to assume with utmost realism what had been experienced and the projections—which interest us—of what has happened vis-à-vis China and its possible ramifications for this region. From this broad, diverse and pluralist reflection, the essays emerged that we have brought together in this book. A reading of them as a whole ratifies the axiom that, on occasion, rings quite true: there are times when the whole is greater than the sum of its parts.

July 2020

II. Peru and Latin America Facing the COVID-19 Pandemic: What can be Learned from China's Experience?

Carlos Aquino[1]

The COVID-19 pandemic has had devastating consequences for the entire world, and for Latin America in particular. The region will be the hardest-hit economically, and will also figure among the countries that will experience the highest rates of contagions and mortality.

The question put forward here is why this is so, and in any case, what can be learned from China's experience and from other Asian countries that have largely managed to control the pandemic, where there have been considerably lower numbers of infected and fatalities. Many of these countries will also experience a lesser negative impact on their economies, especially compared to what will happen to the Latin American countries.

This writing will attempt to answer these questions. It will be divided into five parts: first, the experience of Peru and Latin America with the COVID-19 pandemic; second, what this pandemic teaches from a social and economic perspective; third, the prejudices and errors in the fight against COVID-19 in Latin

1. Coordinator, CEAS.

America; fourth, the perspectives from Peru relative to what China has experienced, what can be learned from China and from others in Asia. Fifth and last, some Conclusions will be presented.

1. The Experience of Peru and Latin America with the COVID-19 Pandemic: Effects on the Number of Infected, Deaths, and on the Economy

The first thing that should be said is that the analysis of the pandemic's effects is somehow partial and incomplete, since the pandemic is still in full swing in many countries, including in Latin America, and has not yet been brought under control in Peru. Thus, things may be more complex than at first glance: the economy may fall lower than projected, and in the case of persons infected and fatalities, clearly over time the numbers will exceed those presented in this chapter.

In any case, as of June 28, 2020, the completion date of this writing, of the 28 countries most affected in terms of number of fatalities and infections, five are Latin American. In terms of numbers of deaths, Brazil is ranked second in the world, Mexico seventh, Peru 11th, Chile 16th, Ecuador 20th, and Colombia 22nd. Brazil is also the country with the second highest number of infected persons in the world, and Peru and Chile figure among the top ten. This figure will almost certainly be higher in

Brazil and Mexico, because unlike countries such as Peru and Chile, the two have not done much testing. Brazil has only tested 1.8 times more than Peru, even though its population is 6.5 times larger; and Mexico has only done half as many tests as Chile, even though its population is 6.7 times larger. (See Table 1.)

Table 1. Indicators for COVID-19 affected countries, by number of deaths, number of infected, and number of tests performed

RCP Coronavirus Tracker

Coronavirus (COVID-19) Global Deaths

Coronavirus (COVID-19) U.S. Deaths

Country	Deaths▾	Deaths / 1M pop▸	New Deaths▸	Tests▸	Estimated Cases▸	Confirmed Cases▸	Confirmed Case Fatality Rate▸	Confirmed Cases / 1M pop▸	Seasonal Flu Deaths' (CDC/WHO 2017)▸
	632,368	-	-	-	-	16,486,197	-	-	-
United States	146,537	447.9	+354	50,897,040	-	4,121,786	3.56%	12,598.4	40,905
Brazil	82,925	395.9	+35	4,911,063	-	2,234,602	3.71%	10,667.9	16,910
United Kingdom	45,554	685.1	+53	13,763,289	-	297,146	15.33%	4,469.1	13,879
Mexico	41,190	326.4	+790	861,852	-	362,274	11.37%	2,870.8	6,075
Italy	35,092	580.7	+10	6,415,041	-	245,338	14.30%	4,059.8	10,058
India	30,601	22.6	+711	15,075,369	-	1,284,638	2.38%	949.7	362,108
France	30,172	450.4	-	2,900,040	-	178,336	16.92%	2,662.2	9,199
Spain	28,429	608.4	+3	6,320,836	-	317,246	8.96%	6,789.8	8,091
Peru	17,455	545.7	-	2,133,175	-	366,550	4.76%	11,458.5	9,212
Iran**	15,074	184.3	+221	2,254,123	-	284,034	5.31%	3,472.3	3,156
Russia	12,892	89.2	+147	26,000,908	-	795,038	1.62%	5,502.8	18,654
Belgium	9,808	858.7	+3	1,501,396	-	64,627	15.18%	5,658.1	2,662
Germany	9,183	110.7	+1	7,418,812	-	204,570	4.49%	2,466.8	16,876
Canada	8,870	239.3	-	3,659,778	-	112,240	7.90%	3,028.7	4,569
Chile	8,722	465.7	-	1,445,773	-	336,402	2.59%	17,961.4	2,235
Colombia	7,373	148.5	-	1,292,501	-	218,428	3.38%	4,399.5	2,527
Netherlands	6,139	356.3	-	851,885	-	52,404	11.71%	3,041.3	2,312
South Africa	5,940	102.8	-	2,585,474	-	394,948	1.50%	6,835.4	8,409
Pakistan	5,709	26.9	+32	1,799,290	-	269,191	2.12%	1,268.5	42,650
Sweden	5,667	556.5	-	751,213	-	78,504	7.22%	7,709.2	1,541
Turkey	5,545	67.4	-	4,403,031	-	222,402	2.49%	2,701.7	5,613
Ecuador	5,418	317.1	-	213,002	-	77,257	7.01%	4,522.1	1,444
China*	4,634	3.3	-	90,410,000	-	83,729	5.53%	60.1	91,814
Indonesia	4,576	17.1	+117	1,310,924	-	93,657	4.89%	349.9	59,453
Egypt	4,440	45.1	-	135,000	-	89,745	4.95%	911.8	22,843
Iraq	4,122	107.2	+80	861,165	-	102,226	4.03%	2,659.8	8,113
Bangladesh	2,801	17.4	+50	1,079,007	-	216,110	1.30%	1,339.3	36,590
Saudi Arabia	2,635	78.2	+34	2,894,426	-	260,394	1.01%	7,726.8	1,974
Argentina	2,617	58.8	+29	593,044	-	141,900	1.84%	3,189.2	7,156
Bolivia	2,328	205.1	+55	139,337	-	64,135	3.63%	5,649.1	3,159

Source: See website of RealClear Politics: RCP Coronavirus Tracker: Viewed on 28-06-2020.https://www.realclearpolitics.com/coronavirus/?fbclid=IwAR0Z-gG-ghP_Xp9rXMPN07ji- PIisIr_dggoLyDaUSYg1k27aqqMS3YTt8n0w

Also shown in Table 1, Chile and Peru have the highest number globally of infected persons per million inhabitants; Chile is in first place with 14,296.7, and Peru in second place with 8,627.6.

However, in terms of economic impact, the Latin American region will be the hardest hit worldwide. According to World Bank projections published on June 8, 2020, the region's economy will likely fall by 7.2% year-on-year by 2020, compared to the world average of a 5.2% drop. (See Table 2.)

Table 2. Real GDP (variation with respect to the year before)

	2017	2018	2019	2020	2021
World	3.3	3.0	2.4	-5.2	4.2
Advanced economies	2.5	2.1	1.6	-7.0	3.9
United States	2.4	2.9	2.3	-6.1	4.0
Euro Area	2.5	1.9	1.2	-9.1	4.5
Japan	2.2	0.3	0.7	-6.1	2.5
Emerging market and developing economies	4.5	4.3	3.5	-2.5	4.6
Commodity-exporting EMDEs	2.2	2.1	1.5	-4.8	3.1
Other EMDEs	6.1	5.7	4.8	-1.1	5.5
Other EMDEs excluding China	5.4	4.8	3.2	-3.6	3.6
East Asia and Pacific	6.5	6.3	5.9	0.5	6.6
China	6.8	6.6	6.1	1.0	6.9
Indonesia	5.1	5.2	5.0	0.0	4.8
Thailand	4.1	4.2	2.4	-5.0	4.1
Europe and Central Asia	4.1	3.3	2.2	-4.7	3.6
Russia	1.8	2.5	1.3	-6.0	2.7
Turkey	7.5	2.8	0.9	-3.8	5.0
Poland	4.9	5.3	4.1	-4.2	2.8
Latin America and the Caribbean	1.9	1.7	0.8	-7.2	2.8
Brazil	1.3	1.3	1.1	-8.0	2.2
Mexico	2.1	2.2	-0.3	-7.5	3.0
Argentina	2.7	-2.5	-2.2	-7.3	2.1
Middle East and North Africa	1.1	0.9	-0.2	-4.2	2.3
Saudi Arabia	-0.7	2.4	0.3	-3.8	2.5
Iran	3.8	-4.7	-8.2	-5.3	2.1
Egypt	4.2	5.3	5.6	3.0	2.1
South Asia	6.5	6.5	4.7	-2.7	2.8
India	7.0	6.1	4.2	-3.2	3.1
Pakistan	5.2	5.5	1.9	-2.6	-0.2
Bangladesh	7.3	7.9	8.2	1.6	1.0
Sub-Saharan Africa	2.6	2.6	2.2	-2.8	3.1
Nigeria	0.8	1.9	2.2	-3.2	1.7
South Africa	1.4	0.8	0.2	-7.1	2.9
Angola	-0.1	-2.0	-0.9	-4.0	3.1

Source: World Bank: "Global Economic Prospects", June 2020, page 4.

The World Bank study shows that of the total of 42 emerging and developing economies (i.e., excluding the advanced economies) whose growth may fall by more than 5% year-on-year in 2020, 15 will be in Latin America (i.e., practically half of the countries in the region). Of the 19 countries considered to be emerging and developing economies and whose economies are expected this year to fall by more than 7% year-on-year, eight are in the Latin American region-nearly half of the group, or nearly one-fourth of the countries in the region. (See Table 3, the forecast for the countries of the region, excluding Cuba and Venezuela.)

Table 3. Projections for the Latin American and Caribbean countries (Real GDP growth at market prices)

	2017	2018	2019e	2020f	2021f
Argentina	2.7	-2.5	-2.2	-7.3	2.1
Belize	1.9	2.1	0.3	-13.5	8.7
Bolivia	4.2	4.2	2.7	-5.9	2.2
Brazil	1.3	1.3	1.1	-8.0	2.2
Chile	1.3	3.9	1.1	-4.3	3.1
Colombia	1.4	2.5	3.3	-4.9	3.6
Costa Rica	3.9	2.7	2.1	-3.3	3.0
Dominica	-9.5	0.5	9.6	-4.0	4.0
Dominican Republic	4.7	7.0	5.1	-0.8	2.5
Ecuador	2.4	1.3	0.1	-7.4	4.1
El Salvador	2.3	2.4	2.4	-5.4	3.6
Grenada	4.4	4.2	3.1	-9.6	6.5
Guatemala	3.0	3.1	3.6	-3.0	4.1
Guyana	2.1	4.1	4.7	51.1	8.1
Haiti	1.2	1.5	-0.9	-3.5	1.0
Honduras	4.8	3.7	2.7	-5.8	3.7
Jamaica	1.0	1.9	0.7	-6.2	2.7
Mexico	2.1	2.2	-0.3	-7.5	3.0
Nicaragua	4.6	4.0	-3.9	-6.3	0.7
Panama	5.6	3.7	3.0	-2.0	4.2
Paraguay	5.0	3.4	0.0	-2.8	4.2
Peru	2.5	4.0	2.2	-12.0	7.0
St. Lucia	2.2	1.4	1.4	-8.8	8.3
St. Vincent and the Grenadines	1.0	2.0	0.4	-5.5	1.0
Suriname	1.8	2.6	2.3	-5.0	3.0
Uruguay	2.6	1.6	0.2	-3.7	4.6

Source: World Bank: "Global Economic Prospects", June 2020, p. 86.

Finally, it should be said that two of the three economies

that may record the worst performance in 2020 worldwide are in Latin America-Peru and Belize. Belize is expected to have the worst performance-its economy may fall-13.5% year-on-year. The second worst (-13.0%) could be the South Asian country of Maldives, and the third, Peru (-12.0%). In a report published by the IMF on June 24, 2020, the projections for Latin America's economy were even gloomier. It was foreseen that the region would record a year-to-year drop of-9.4%, the worst among the developing economies. (See Table 4.)

Table 4. Latest growth projections from World Economic Outlook

(real GDP, annual percent change)	2019	PROJECTIONS 2020	2021
World Output	2.9	-4.9	5.4
Advanced Economies	1.7	-8.0	4.8
United States	2.3	-8.0	4.5
Euro Area	1.3	-10.2	6.0
Germany	0.6	-7.8	5.4
France	1.5	-12.5	7.3
Italy	0.3	-12.8	6.3
Spain	2.0	-12.8	6.3
Japan	0.7	-5.8	2.4
United Kingdom	1.4	-10.2	6.3
Canada	1.7	-8.4	4.9
Other Advanced Economies	1.7	-4.8	4.2
Emerging Markets and Developing Economies	3.7	-3.0	5.9
Emerging and Developing Asia	5.5	-0.8	7.4
China	6.1	1.0	8.2
India	4.2	-4.5	6.0
ASEAN 5	4.9	-2.0	6.2
Emerging and Developing Europe	2.1	-5.8	4.3
Russia	1.3	-6.6	4.1
Latin America and the Caribbean	0.1	-9.4	3.7
Brazil	1.1	-9.1	3.6
Mexico	-0.3	-10.5	3.3
Middle East and Central Asia	1.0	-4.7	3.3
Saudi Arabia	0.3	-6.8	3.1
Sub-Saharan Africa	3.1	-3.2	3.4
Nigeria	2.2	-5.4	2.6
South Africa	0.2	-8.0	3.5
Low-Income Developing Countries	5.2	-1.0	5.2

Source: "Reopening from the Great Lockdown: Uneven and Uncertain recovery" June 24, 2020 .

On June 26, the IMF published the growth projections for Latin America, for some of the countries in greater detail. (See Table 5.) As the table indicates, the outlook is quite bleak. It is projected that several countries will experience a fall in annual growth of more than 10% in 2020. A reduction of Peru's GDP ofnearly 14% is expected, according to this projection.

Table 5. Outlook for the Latin American countries (Real GDP growth, percentages)

	2018	2019	Proyecciones 2020	2021	Diferencia respecto a proyecciones de informe WEO de abril de 2020 2020	2021
América Latina y el Caribe	1.1	0.1	-9.4	3.7	-4.2	0.3
Excluida Venezuela	1.8	0.8	-9.2	3.9	-4.2	0.4
América del Sur²	0.4	-0.1	-9.5	3.9	-4.4	0.5
Excluida Venezuela	1.4	1.0	-9.2	4.2	-4.4	0.6
CAPRD³	3.9	3.2	-5.9	3.2	-3.5	-0.8
El Caribe						
Dependientes del turismo⁴	1.9	1.2	-10.3	4.8	-2.8	-1.0
Exportadores de materias primas⁴	0.7	0.9	3.5	3.2	-1.9	-0.4
América Latina						
Argentina	-2.5	-2.2	-9.9	3.9	-4.2	-0.5
Brasil	1.3	1.1	-9.1	3.6	-3.8	0.7
Chile	3.9	1.1	-7.5	5.0	-3.0	-0.3
Colombia	2.5	3.3	-7.8	4.0	-5.4	0.3
México	2.2	-0.3	-10.5	3.3	-3.9	0.3
Perú	4.0	2.2	-13.9	6.5	-9.4	1.3

Fuentes: Base de datos de *Perspectivas de la economía mundial* del FMI y cálculos del personal técnico.
1/ CAPRD = Centroamérica, Panamá y la República Dominicana.
2/ Excluye Guyana y Suriname.
3/ Incluye Antigua y Barbuda, Aruba, Las Bahamas, Barbados, Belice, Dominica, Granada, Jamaica, Saint Kitts y Nevis, San Vicente y las Granadinas y Santa Lucia.
4/ Incluye Guyana, Suriname y Trinidad y Tobago.

Source: FMI [IMF] Blog: "Perspectivas para America Latina y el Caribe: La pandemia se intensifica", 26 de junio del 2020.

2. Lessons of the pandemic from a social and economic perspective

It is worth asking why Peru and Latin America have had such a disappointing social and economic behavior in the face of the pandemic. This is important to ascertain because, as we shall see, the pandemic is revealing many of the region's deficiencies that will need to be resolved in order to face a possible similar situation in the future. This is an imperative in any case, for the region to achieve a more balanced and egalitarian social and economic development.

From the societal point of view, several problems can be discerned:

(a) The region has one of the greatest income inequalities in the world.[2] The percentage of poverty in the population is also high, and the pandemic will render this situation more critical. According to an ECLAC report dated April 21, 2020, the poverty level will rise from 30.3% to 34.7% in 2020.[3] Those who can

2. According to the ECLAC Executive Secretary, it is the largest in the world. See Diario El Espectador: "Latinoamérica, el continente ms desigual del mundo: CEPAL"https://www.elespectador.com/eco- nomia/latinoamérica-el-continente-mas-desigual-del-mundo-cepal-articulo-903452/

3. See Agencia EFE: "Cepal: La pandemia provocara la peor recesión en la historia de Latinoa- mérica"https://www.efe.com/efe/américa/economia/cepal-la-pandemia-provocara-peor-rece-sion-en-historia-de-latinoamérica/20000011-4227121

afford to do so can access the private health system and circumvent the pandemic, while most of the population must depend on the public health system, which in many countries of the region is quite precarious. The public health system has collapsed in many of the countries. Since early May, in provinces of Peru such as Loreto, one of the poorest in the country, there was no longer any oxygen or equipment for Intensive Care Units (ICUs). However, since the beginning of June this situation had begun to be felt in Lima, the capital city, and as of June 24 it was reported that the public health system in Lima had collapsed.[4] The spectacle of many people buying oxygen with their own means, as began to be seen in early June in the capital, was quite dramatic, showing as it did that the state was incapable of providing such an essential good as oxygen during the pandemic.[5]

(b) The Latin American countries have weak social safety nets. When people lose their jobs they have no unemployment insurance and are left without an income. This is what happened in the quarantines implanted in many countries. And despite the fact that various countries implemented a system of money transfers for a certain percentage of the population, when the quarantine period was lengthened the subsidies were insufficient

4. See newspaper El Comercio, 24 de junio, p. 3: "Personal del Rebagliati asegura que ya no quedan camas UCI" http://elcomercio.peruquiosco.pe/m/a/20200624/3 .
5. See CNN website: "Peruvians cry out for oxygen as coronavirus takes its toll" https://edition.cnn. com/2020/06/05/américas/peru-coronavirus-oxygen-shortages-intl/index.html.

and people went out to the streets to earn a little income. In Peru's case, for example, a state of emergency was declared on the 16th of March and extended until the 30th of June (which restricted many activities, especially in the first two months). In spite of the government's beginning to grant subsidies to a significant percentage of families, because of the quarantine's duration this money was insufficient. Peru is implementing one of the most ambitious programs for delivering subsidies to the Latin American population. The government plan is to provide a sum of money, equivalent to around 220 dollars, to seven million families out of a total of nine million in the country. Even the finance minister announced on June 25 that the provision of an additional amount was under study for the neediest families.[6] However, there are various problems with this scheme. More than three-and-a-half months after the pandemic began, the subsidy has still not been received by all seven million families. The disbursements led to crowding in the banks, where it is said that contagion occurred. Many families have been left without the bonus because they were not included the list of beneficiaries that was prepared based on the 2017[7] National Census (and the economic situation of many people is alleged to have changed between that date and the present). It seems clear that the bonus

6. See newspaper Gestión: "MEF evalúa entregar más bonos para hogares vulnerables".

7. See Tikitakas website: "Bono Familiar Universal: Cómo se ha armado el padrón de los beneficiados?" https://peru.as.com/peru/2020/04/28/tikitakas/1588088925_704007. html.

has turned out to be insufficient, given the long duration of the quarantine imposed by the government. What should have been done from the beginning was to transfer to all recipients a sum of money for covering their basic needs, and thus enable the implementation of a strict quarantine, which would have reduced the numbers of infected and deaths, and shortened the quarantine period, preventing a greater negative impact on the economy.[8] On the other hand, many Latin American governments have demonstrated inefficiency in their actions and there have been cases of corruption, including irregularities in handling the funds allocated to combating the pandemic.[9] From the economic point of view, several problems can also be pointed out, summarized here in the following two points:

First, a significant percentage of the region's economy is informal, wherein many people work without a fixed income, and if they do not work one day then they will not have any earnings for that day. This is why they do not have savings either for coping with a quarantine that has disrupted the country's economic activities and has forced people to remain in their

8. As some economists have requested. See for example my Blog of March 22, 2020, Carlos Aquino, Blog Asia Pacifico: "El impacto en la economía peruana del neo coronavirus y que hacer" https://asiapacifico-carlosaquino.blogspot.com/2020/03/el-impacto-en-la-economia-

9. See Gestión Newspaper: "El coronavirus favorece la pandemia de la corrupción en Latinoamérica" https://gestion.pe/mundo/el-coronavirus-favorece-la-pandemia-de-la-corrupcion-en-latinoaméri- News

homes, as has happened in most of the Latin American countries. This is precisely the reason offered to explain why the Peruvian economy will suffer such a big fall this year, why unemployment has risen so much and the poverty level will rise at year's end. It also explains the high number of infected and deaths in various countries of the region, such as in Peru.[10] It is said that in Peru's case, perhaps 60% or even 70% of the people work in the informal sector;[11] thus, despite the quarantine, many people went out to seek some income and this allowed the infections to continue increasing.

Second, many economies in the region are increasingly dependent on the external market, whether for export earnings, tourism, foreign direct investment or remittances. With the stoppage of economic activity that occurred in all countries of the world during the first months of 2020, income from these sources will fall abruptly. In exports, if we examine Peru, for example, exports of goods in 2019 equaled 20.3% of its GDP and totaled US$ 47.688 billion dollars.[12] With the world economy falling

10. See Time, "Peru Locked Down Hard and Early. Why Is Its Coronavirus Outbreak So Bad" https://time.com/5844768/peru-coronavirus/

11. See World Economic Forum website: "The plight of Peru illustrates the danger of COVID-19 https://www.weforum.org/agenda/2020/06/the-plight-of-peru-illus-trates-the-danger-of-covid-19-to-eveloping-countries?fbclid=IwAR2QWHHOclMEq01tA-VUNY9D7TxAbnPsxR2XwTzvXNTdr_NYQFzBdhw9KkrY

12. See Banco Central de Reserva del Perú: "Indicadores Económicos I trimestre 2020" https://www.bcrp.gob.pe/docs/Estadisticas/indicadores-trimestrales.pdf www.bcrp.gob.pe/docs/Estadisticas/indicadores-trimestrales.pdf

5.2% in 2020 according to the World Bank, or 4.9% according to the IMF, this sector's prospects are not favorable. The World Trade Organization's best-case scenario is that trade volume in 2020 will fall 13% (or 32% in the worst-case scenario).[13] In addition, in countries such as Mexico that depend heavily on a single market as an export destination, the scenario will be worse. Mexico sends 80% of its export goods to the U.S., and as shown in Tables 2 and 4, will experience a drop in its economy of 7% or 8% year-on-year, respectively. In addition, most Latin American countries depend primarily on the export of raw materials and many of these will register price drops. For countries like Venezuela that depend almost exclusively on oil and whose product has experienced a drastic price drop, the situation will be even more critical. With respect to tourism revenues, as shown in Table 5, tourism-dependent countries in the region will see a 10.3% fall in their year-on-year GDP in 2020. Even Mexico, a country that also takes in considerable revenues from the other sources mentioned such as exports, foreign direct investment and remittances, tourism revenues accounted for 17.2% of its GDP in 2018.[14] With most of the world quarantined during the first half of 2020, the prospects of tourism reaching a level anywhere

13. See WTO: "Trade falls steeply in first half of 2020" https://www.wto.org/english/news_e/pres20_e/pr858_e.htm

14. "Who depends the most on tourists": http://www.gzeromedia. com/the-graphic-truth-who-depends-the-most-on-tourists

close to the 2019 levels are nil. Regarding foreign investment (Inversión extranjera directa, IED), Peru for example received investments for US$ 8.9 billion in 2019, representing 3.8% of its GDP. However, in 2020 this income is expected to fall by 82.5% according to the projections of the country's Central Reserve Bank, or Banco Central de Reserva.[15] With the world economy in a recession in 2020, it would be logical for the FDI to likewise experience a significant fall in the same year. And on the subject of remittances, there are countries that are heavily dependent on this income source. For example, in 2018, the remittances to Haiti from citizens abroad accounted for 32.5% of its GDP; to El Salvador, 20.7%; and to Honduras, 19.9%.[16] The remittances are sent from developed countries such as in North America and Europe, and as shown in Tables 2 and 4, the economies of these countries will be the hardest hit in the world; thus, remittances should also experience a drastic drop in 2020. For example, IMF projections are that the US economy will fall by 8% year-on-year in 2020 and that the Eurozone countries will see their economies fall by 10.2% year-on-year.

Biases and Errors in Latin America's fight against

15. See newspaper Diario Gestión p. 10, 23 de junio del 2020: "BCR prevé que inversión extranjera directa caería 82.5% en el 2020"

16. See GZERO website: "Who depends the most on tourists" https://www.gzeromedia.com/the- graphic-truth-who-depends-the-most-on-tourists

Covid-19

Some mistakes made in the fight against the pandemic that can be synthesized in just two are the following:

First is that, unfortunately, some governments seemed unable to understand the magnitude of the problem and even now apparently still fail to grasp it. Brazil and Mexico, the two countries most hard hit as well, initially hesitated to implement measures against the pandemic because of the position held by their top leaders of minimizing Covid-19, treating it like a simple cold.[17] To this day the president of Brazil considers it so, and even filed an appeal against the order issued by a Brazilian court that he wear a mask at public events.[18]

Second, there have also been cases of discrimination, for example at some point against people of Asian origin or against the medical personnel who were providing treatment to victims of the pandemic.[19] There is also considerable disinformation, as in other regions, regarding the pandemic's origin, or remedies or

17. See CNN website: "Why are these three Presidents downplaying coronavirus warnings?" ht- tps://edition.cnn.com/2020/03/24/américas/coronavirus-latin-américa-presidents-intl/index. html

18. See France 24 website: "Brazil`s Bolsonaro appeals court order on wearing mask" https://www. france24.com/en/20200626-brazil-s-bolsonaro-appeals-court-order-on-wearing-mask

19. See DW News website: "Especial Coronavirus: prejuicios y discriminación" https://www. dw.com/es/especial-coronavirus-prejuicios-y-desinformaci%C3%B3n/av-53429667

possible cures that are being touted. Especially in social networks this has become common with the circulation of so-called "fake news."

Peru's perspective on China's experience and what can be learned from China and Asia in general

Surprisingly, the figures for deaths and infections in the Asian region (in this article we will refer in particular to the countries and economies of East Asia) have been quite low, especially in comparison to those of the Latin American countries. Not only this, but the impact on their economies is allegedly not as severe as what is being experienced by most Latin American countries. As Table 1 shows, China, the first epicenter of the pandemic, ranks 19th in the world in number of deaths, and Indonesia ranks 23rd. The same source indicates that the Philippines ranks 34th, and countries such as Japan and South Korea, geographically located very close to China and that maintain a close relationship with her, for example in business and tourism, only rank 37th and 60th, respectively. If we consider the death toll per million inhabitants in Brazil, the figure is 272.8; 209.1 in Mexico; 285.6 in Peru; 285.5 in Chile and 259 in Ecuador-the countries most affected in Latin America. But in East Asia these numbers are much lower. In China the number of deaths per million inhabitants is 3.3; in Indonesia, 10.3; in the Philippines, 11.7; in Japan, 7.7; and in

South Korea just 5.4. As for Vietnam, it has null deaths according to its official statistics.[20] It should be recalled that a large number of these Asian countries have already brought the epidemic under control, while the Latin American countries have not (although there is always the danger, in Asia and worldwide, of a second wave of contagion). The above is interesting because these Asian countries have large populations, several of them have small territories, are densely populated and quite urbanized. Not just this, but China is in close geographical proximity to them, there are strong commercial ties between them and large numbers of Chinese tourists visit these countries. Despite which they have largely managed to control the pandemic with fewer numbers of infected and deaths. In terms of numbers of infected, for example, none of these countries are among the top 20 worldwide.

Why is this? One could mention several reasons that could serve as lessons for Latin America:

First, these countries acted quickly to control the contagion. Initially, after China declared the quarantine on January 23 in Wuhan City, where the first massive spread of contagion was reported, these countries began controlling the entry of potentially infected persons. For instance, Vietnam is said to have begun implementing health controls by January 11 in response to the events in China, even before the Wuhan quarantine began, by

20. See website of RealClear Politics: RCP Coronavirus Tracker: Taken on 06-28-2020 https://www.realclearpolitics.com/coronavirus/?fbclid=IwAR0ZgG-ghP_Xp9rXMPN07jiPIisIr_dg- goLyDaUSYg1k27aqqMS3YTt8n0w

tracking the temperatures of passengers in airports,[21] for example.

Second, they implemented policies to effectively isolate the initially infected, and to test those suspected of being infected. Quarantine in the Northeast Asian countries and economies was not always total, except in China and Vietnam, but the governments' call to the populace to stay home and/or restrict their movements was usually observed. In Southeast Asia, like Indonesia and Thailand, there was a mandatory quarantine.

Third, these countries, especially in Northeast Asia, tried to assist their populations, who also saw a reduction of their incomes due to restrictions on economic activity, through subsidies.

The most generous have been Japan[22] and South Korea, which have distributed bonuses to practically their entire populations to mitigate income loss and the consequent fall in consumption and demand, and general decline of their economies.

Fourth, it could be argued that China, Japan, South Korea, for example, have more economic resources than many countries in Latin America, and this is true, as they are more developed countries with per capita income in China, for example, of US$10,000 per year, and in South Korea, two and a half times this level, and in Japan, four times as high as that of China. But

---

21. See World Economic Forum website: "Here are 4 ways Viet Nam has managed to control CO- VID-19" https://www.weforum.org/agenda/2020/05/vietnam-control-covid-19/

22. See SCMP website: "Coronavirus: Japan to give each resident US$930 as pandemic batters economy" https://www.scmp.com/news/asia/east-asia/article/3080493/coronavirus-japan-give-all-residents-stimulus-payments-us930

countries like Indonesia have an income level that is similar to or lower than those of several Latin American countries, and Vietnam has a lower per capita income than most countries in the region. The annual income in Vietnam is less than one-third that of Brazil and less than half that of Peru; however, as mentioned above, according to official figures Vietnam has had zero deaths from COVID-19.[23]

Fifth, as Vietnam's case also illustrates, in East Asia various countries successfully mobilized their populations by recruiting them as volunteers, or the state mobilized all of its resources to effectively control the pandemic. In many of these countries the state enjoys legitimacy and is seen as relatively efficient, and its directives are largely followed. They are efficient and have low levels of corruption, especially if compared to many Latin American countries.

Sixth, it can also be pointed out that several East Asian countries made extensive use of technology to combat the pandemic. China deployed the almost all of the tools she has been able to develop in recent years, in informatics and communications, that have enabled her to be one of the most advanced countries in these fields, if not the most advanced. For example, China was able to track the cases of infected people, control the movements

23. See VOA website: "How did become Vietnam biggest nation without coronavirus deaths" https://www.voanews.com/covid-19-pandemic/how-did-vietnam-become-biggest-nation-without-coronavirus-deaths

of the population (through the installation of health applications in peoples' phones),[24] use drones to deliver food and medicines, warn people to comply with health standards, etc.[25] It is said that over 80% of the Chinese population has access to smartphones that allow the installation of these applications. Also, the use of digital money, of a delivery system for purchases, and other media that allow maintaining "social distancing" and prevent contagion (all areas wherein China is the most advanced in the world), enabled her to control the pandemic relatively quickly. The fact that China is quite advanced in 5G Internet technology is what has also allowed her to apply all the above, areas in which Latin American countries are lagging behind China. As for the impact on their economies, as indicated by the forecasts of both the World Bank and the IMF, the East Asian region is expected to be the least affected in the world. Table 2 shows that East Asia, grouped under East Asian and Pacific economies, would have a year-on-year growth rate of just 0.5% in 2020. Table 4 presents the IMF forecasts with East Asia grouped under Emerging and Developing Asia. These economies are expected to decline by 0.8% year-on-year in 2020, which, while negative,

24. See Business Insider: "As China lifts its coronavirus lockdowns, authorities are using a co- lor-coded health system to dictate where citizens can go. Here`s how it works" https://www.bu- sinessinsider.com/coronavirus-china-health-software-color-coded-how-it-works-2020-4

25. See ITN website: "Deployment of Health IT in China`s fight against the COVID-19 pandemics"https://www.itnonline.com/article/deployment-health-it-china%E2%80%99s-fight-against-covid-19-pandemic

still comparesquite favorably with the Latin American countries, whose economies are expected to decline 9.4% year-on-year.

Conclusions

The COVID-19 pandemic has inflicted a terrible toll on the Latin American countries in terms of numbers of infected and deaths, and will plunge the economies into a deep recession in 2020. The deficiencies in the social and economic systems of these countries and in the actions adopted by their governments in response to the pandemic can be seen as the main causes of this. There have also been errors made and prejudices that have harmed and blocked the fight against the pandemic. However, the East Asian region, and China in particular, whose populations and economies have suffered less, can offer various lessons to Latin America. One of these is the need to have a more efficient state so that it can act quickly in response to these emergencies, have more widespread social safety nets, use information and communications technologies, etc. In summary, there is quite a lot to be learned from Asia to be able to tackle future emergencies such as COVID-19 and to be able to achieve sustained growth with more equality. It must be remembered that the Asian economies have grown the most in the recent past, they are growing the most at present, and they will grow the most in the foreseeable future. Especially in the coming post-pandemic period, they will be the first to recover. Here China's role is especially significant. China has been the engine of the world economy since the early years of this century and the countries of Latin America have benefited from the Asian giant's great demand for their raw materials. In this pandemic, China has been the first economy to recover and is likewise expected to be able to contribute to the recovery of the rest of the economies, such as those of Latin America. In addition, China has offered assistance to many countries in dealing with the pandemic, whether through medical equipment and supplies or by sending medical personnel. It is therefore hoped that Latin America and China can continue to strengthen not just their economic ties, but also their bonds of cooperation. China is already the biggest trading partner of several countries in the region, she is the second largest regional partner after the U.S., she is a major foreign investor and lender, and 19 countries in the region have adhered to The Belt and Road Initiative.

III. The Covid-19 Pandemic's Impacts on Chinese-Latin American Relations: The Case of Argentina

Dr. Jorge E. Malena[1]

Abstract

Since March 2020, the majority of the Latin American nations have been the recipients of considerable health and medical aid from China in order to cope with the Covid-19 pandemic. This has implied an impact on China's diplomatic relations with the countries of the region, which, given their geographical location, history and political culture, lie within the U.S.'s sphere of influence. This article analyzes Chinese-Latin American cooperation within the framework of the growing tensions between Washington D.C. and Beijing, with emphasis on the collaboration between China and Argentina in the response to the pandemic. The article concludes with a vision of the future of the international system, and the course that bilateral relations will follow at the national and subcontinental level.

1. Director, Executive Program on Contemporary China, Faculty of Social Sciences, Universidad Católica Argentina (UCA); Coordinator, China Work Group, Argentine Council for International Relations (CARI) China Work Group.

Key Words: China, cooperation, pandemic, Latin America, Argentina.

Introduction

It is written in "The Analects", the compilation of the teachings of Confucius, how Zilu, one of the Master's best-known disciples, asked him about death. The Master said, "You know nothing of life as yet; how then can you know death?" Our lives have been affected by the Covid-19 pandemic and the experience has given us a chance to reflect on life and death.

Why do I mention this? Because while not all events qualify as geopolitical, there are some that can be linked to and even affect the international system, because of the magnitude of their impact. The pandemic is an unprecedented event because of its sweep and danger. We are witnessing how it is affecting people's lives, their sources of employment, means of transportation and global trade on a large scale and with devastating impact.

In light of this, the collective response to the health and medical crisis precipitated by Covid-19 is of central importance. In principle, concretizing said response lies in the hands of intergovernmental entities, with the World Health Organization (WHO) at their helm. The People's Republic of China (hereinafter "PRC") seeks to establish itself as a pole of global cooperation. Because of China's proactive role in the hour of providing aid, the pandemic has stimulated reflection on the PRC's position on the international stage. This position exerts an impact on the Latin American countries, which, by their geographical location, history and political culture, lie within the sphere of influence of the United States (henceforth "U.S.").

Since March of 2020, most of the Latin American nations have received aid from China in order to cope with the Covid-19 pandemic, in the form of health and medical supplies or advice. However, this is not the first time that China has offered aid to the subcontinent. Following the 2008 recession, Beijing financed a global stimulus package, equivalent to 7% of China's gross domestic product (GDP), that enabled it to acquire raw materials from Latin America, such as oil, wood and minerals (Angelo & Chavez, 2020).

The PRC has stood out In the concert of nations for its cooperation initiatives, notwithstanding the statements of certain analysts in the West that China is using health expertise and medical equipment as means for exercising soft power in Latin America, through its development of a "face-mask diplomacy"(Li & Mc Elveen, 2020).[2] China has refuted this concept and made use instead of the term "the Health Silk Road" (Ministerio de RR.EE. de la RPCh, marzo de 2020). This should not be analyzed purely from the perspective of the bid between the Asian giant and the U.S. to expand their respective spheres of influence, but also as a gesture of international cooperation.

2. It is noteworthy that the term was used for the first time by the cited source in early March 2020, with no pejorative connotation. The term was employed on that occasion to highlight the rapprochement between Beijing and Tokyo, through health cooperation in response to the outbreak's spread.

The following work analyzes Sino-Latin American cooperation, with emphasis on the Sino-Argentine link and their consequent cooperation in the face of the pandemic. A look at the future of the international system and the bilateral relationship follows, at the subcontinental as well as the national level.

The Geopolitics of the Virus: Its Impact on Sino-Latin American Ties

Viruses are humanity's common enemy, able to appear at any time and in any place. Scientific evidence leans toward the improbability of the artificial creation or deliberate manipulation of Covid-19. Consequently, to call it the "Wuhan virus" or the "Chinese virus" is nothing other than ignoring scientific research or seeking to malign China. The U.S. intelligence community itself adopted the scientific community's view that Covid-19 was neither man-made nor genetically modified, as stated in a communique of the Office of the Director of National Intelligence in end-April (*Voz de las Américas,* 2020). It is true that the pandemic's initial manifestation was detected in Wuhan, which obliged the Chinese authorities to create a strict containment plan. However the origin itself of this health crisis has yet to be resolved in a scientific manner. Thus the U.S. authorities' anti-China rhetoric merely hinders the relations between Washington and Beijing. Former U.S. ambassador to China, Max Baucus, said in a May 6 CNN interview that his government's statements reminded him of the McCarthy era. "We are entering an era similar to that of Joe McCarthy, when he hounded the 'reds' and attacked communism" (National Review, 2020).

European leaders themselves have expressed disappointment with the U.S. Government. In the same week when the Trump administration banned flights from Europe, the Chinese government sent medical equipment, including masks, ventilators, personal protection equipment and doctors to Italy and Spain. For this reason the G7 countries rejected Washington's request to refer to Covid-19 as "the Wuhan virus", in the final communique of the virtual meeting held in mid-March (Washington Post, 2020).

Latin America has become a focal point of the strategic dispute between the U.S. and the PRC. This is because the economic growth and political protagonism of Beijing has redounded in smooth interlinkages with a region historically ensconced within Washington's sphere of influence. China's ascendancy made it possible for Latin America to forge closer links with the Asian giant, thanks to the complementarity that exists between them: the Chinese economy needs food products and energy to continue its development, while the subcontinent is rich in commodities but lacks capital and technology. In addition, many Chinese companies have achieved overcapacity in their domestic market and now need to invest abroad.

In the face of this reality, Washington has not stood idly by. U.S. Secretary of State Mike Pompeo warned of the "dangers" of Chinese expansionism in the region, which he described as "predatory economic activity" (New York Times, 2018). In a speech that Kimberly Breier, Assistant Secretary of State for the Western Hemisphere, later delivered before the Council of the Americas, she referred to China as as an actor that "too often departs from international standards of respect for transparency, anti-corruption, financial sustainability, labor rights, environmental and local community protection", and when it did so, "its shady practices leave room for corruption, erosion of governance and challenges to state sovereignty" (Americas Society, 2019). In this regard, the report issued by the White House in May of this year, entitled "U.S. Strategic Approach to the People's Republic of China", affirmed that "the policies of the U.S. are designed to protect our interests and empower our institutions to resist the malicious behavior of the Communist Party of China" (Presidencia de los EE.UU., mayo de 2020).

Notwithstanding these criticisms, the reality is that Washington has disengaged from Latin America and has therefore lost presence on the subcontinent. It is only now, upon the announcement that a U.S. citizen will be placed at the head of the Inter-American Development Bank (breaking a traditional formula established since the IDB's founding of having its headquarters in Washington but with a Latin American director), that a policy of return looms on the horizon, albeit with complex confrontational overtones. Through protectionist policies and postponement of trade agreements, the White House has opened the door for China as well as the European Union (hereinafter "the E.U.") to take the lead in matters of agreements with the region. However, China's influence in the subcontinent is not merely economic, since Beijing also seeks to win support for its Belt and Road Initiative and the adoption of its nuclear and 5G technologies. These developments exert a profound strategic influence because they differ from U.S. interests; hence, the backlash from Washington.

China's economic influence on Latin America is greater than that of any other competitor of Washington in contemporary history (for example, Germany or the Soviet Union). Likewise, the Covid-19 pandemic and its consequent health, medical and economic demands have converged with the tensions between Washington and Beijing since 2017. A kind of "virus geopolitics" has emerged that has impacted on the subcontinent's governments. They face the challenge of dealing with the pandemic's health and economic effects, in addition to the dilemma of which international position to adopt: whether to prioritize the traditional alliance with Washington, or to allow the growing ties with China to prevail; adopt a foreign policy equidistant from both poles, or to "play both hands".

The Regional Context: Sino-Latin American Cooperation

Focusing on the milestones of the last five years, in January of 2015 PRC President Xi Jinping met in Beijing with leaders and foreign ministers of the subcontinent during the First Ministerial Meeting of the China Forum and the Community of Latin American and Caribbean States (*Comunidad de Estados Latinoamericanos y Caribeños*, hereinafter "CELAC"). At the meeting, both parties agreed on a five-year cooperation plan that will encompass policymaking, security, trade, investment, finance, infrastructure, energy, resources, industry, agriculture, science and people-to-people exchanges (*Ministerio de RR.EE. de la RPCh*, 2015).

In 2016 Beijing issued its second White Paper on Latin America relations in which it declares that China seeks to strengthen cooperation based on "equality and mutual benefit" in several key areas, including exchanges and dialog, commerce and investment, agriculture, energy, infrastructure, industry and technological innovation. The White Paper establishes that China "will actively pursue military exchanges and cooperation with Latin America and the Caribbean," and likewise emphasizes that China "does not aim to exclude a third State" *(Ministerio de*

RR.EE. de la RPCh, 2016).

At a second ministerial meeting of the China-CELAC Forum held in January 2018, both parties agreed on an updated plan of cooperation extended until 2021. China also invited the Latin American countries to participate in its Belt and Road Initiative, focused on infrastructure development in various regions around the world. As of end-June 2020, 19 Latin American and Caribbean countries have adhered to the Initiative (Congressional Research Service, 2020).

Total trade between China and Latin America rose from US$ 17 billion in 2002 to nearly US$ 315 billion in 2019. In 2015, President Xi set the goal of increasing total bilateral trade to US$ 500 billion in ten years. PRC acquisitions of goods in Latin America and the Caribbean rose to nearly US$ 165 billion in 2019, representing close to 7.9% of China's total imports. Exports in 2019 from the PRC to the region totaled US$ 142 billion, equivalent to 6% of China's total sales (Congressional Research Service, 2020).

The PRC has become Latin America's second most important trading partner. In Brazil, Argentina, Chile and Peru it has displaced the U.S. from its top position. Regarding credit, China's loans to the subcontinent (mainly for energy and have infrastructure projects) have exceeded the figures provided by the World Bank and the Inter-American Development Bank. This development assistance from Beijing has given access to critical financing to under-resourced, highly indebted governments that must cope with social demands for paved roads, modern public transport and improved services (Angelo & Chavez, 2020).

The PRC's investments in Latin America and the Caribbean for 2005-2019 totaled US$ 130 billion. Energy sector projects accounted for 56% of total investment, while investments in metals and mining accounted for 28%. Chinese investment in construction projects in the region amounted to US$ 61 billion, 53% of which was allocated to energy infrastructure and 27% to transportation (Congressional Research Service, 2020). With respect to the finance sector, Chinese entities such as the Banco de Desarrollo and Export-Import Bank have become the largest lenders of the Latin American states. Total lending amounted to US$ 137 billion between 2005 and 2019, with Venezuela, Brazil, Ecuador and Argentina as the main credit recipients. The majority of the loans (67%) were for energy projects, and 20% for infrastructure projects. Compared to loans from major international financial institutions, these loans are typically granted under less stringent terms and are not subject to political conditionalities or strict environmental guidelines (Congressional Research Service, 2020).

A stark contrast is observed between expanding Sino-Latin American relations and the U.S. government's recent decisions. The Trump administration not only cut back funding for the WHO from US$ 123 million to US$ 58 million for fiscal year 2021, but also followed through on the reduction it had announced for fiscal year 2021 of its contribution to the Pan-American Health Organization (PAHO) from US$ 66 million to US$ 16 million. Let us remember that PAHO is the regional public health agency commissioned with the prevention and containment of outbreaks of communicable diseases in the Americas (U.S. Senate Budget Committee, 2020).

In early April of 2020, President Trump announced during one of his daily coronavirus briefings that he would increase military deployment in the Caribbean and the Eastern Pacific to support anti-drug trafficking missions (US Southern Command, 2020). In the context of a humanitarian crisis, deploying the U.S. Navy and the Coast Guard to ocean zones in close proximity to the shores of nations in need of humanitarian aid can be disconcerting for some government authorities and sectors of public opinion in the subcontinent.

The administration's posture did not stop there. In mid-April this year, the Federal Customs and Border Protection Agency blocked the exit of personal protective equipment and ventilators purchased by Caribbean countries from U.S. vendors. Likewise, the U.S. Navy hospital ship USNS Comfort, which has provided emergency medical assistance on many occasions to Latin American and Caribbean countries, was unable to do so this time since it had to provide assistance to New York City hospitals (Charles & Harris, 2020).

Ties between China and Argentina: Cooperation during the Pandemic

Argentina is the third largest economy in Latin America. Since 2014, the PRC and Argentina have acknowledged each other as "integral strategic partners", as reflected in their ongoing consultations and cooperation in international, scientific and defense matters. Since 2007 there has been increasing investment in various sectors of Argentina's economy (solar energy for example), in excess of US$ 17 billion (Diálogo Inter Americano, 2019).

With regard to trade, China is also the primary importer of Argentine soy and meat. In April 2020 China became Argentina's number one trading partner, moving Brazil to second place. In the same month Argentina exported products to China totaling US$ 509 million, especially soy and meat, exceeding by 50% its exports for the same period in 2019, while exports to Brazil totaled US$ 387 million, showing a fall of 57.3% with respect to the same period in 2019 (Megatrade Virtual, 2020).[3]

The main products of trade on the Argentine side are

3. Argentina and Brazil's trade balance was affected in the leading sector of their bilateral trade, which is motor vehicles and automotive parts. Border restrictions caused by the pandemic resulted in around 10,000 Brazilian-made vehicles being held at the Brazil-Argentina border and forced to wait for authorization for entry into Argentina. Observers complained that Brazil had not resolved its health policy vis-à-vis the pandemic, hence the trade slowdown (Megatrade Virtual, 2020).

agricultural commodities, with a significant increase observed in meat exports. According to Emma Fontanet, International Trade Promotion Manager of Fundación ICBC, compensated beef is sold to China as opposed to steers or loin cuts, plus poultry (chickens). However, according to the expert, prawns are the star commodity. Products purchased from China are mainly technological: mobile phones, power generation sets, devices, semiconductors, automatic machines and chemicals for different industries (Bestani, 2020).

Following the February Covid-19 outbreak in China, Argentine President Alberto Fernández contacted PRC President Xi Jinping to offer his support. In March 2020 the Chinese president replied to President Fernández, advocating the deepening of the ties between the two states. And in mid-March, Chinese ambassador to Argentina, Zou Xiaoli, paid a visit to President Fernández, bringing an offer of a donation of masks, protective goggles, gloves, rapid reagent kits and thermal cameras, as an initial aid consignment (Télam, 17/3/20).

Luo Zhaohui, Chinese Vice Minister of Foreign Affairs, stated during a press conference in Beijing on March 16 that the PRC "will brave the storm together with the peoples of other countries, strengthen cooperation and strive to win the fight against the virus" (Koop et al., 2020). Towards the end of March, at the Extraordinary Meeting of G20 Leaders, President Alberto Fernández suggested that "to deal with this crisis...we must draft and sign a great Global Solidarity Pact. Nothing will be the same after this tragedy. We need to act together immediately, because it is evident that no one can save themselves alone". Keeping to this vision, [President Fernández] held exchanges with several presidents, among them President Xi Jinping (Télam, 26/3/20).

A report was later issued by the Chinese Embassy in Buenos Aires on the donations that had been made, including the reference to a mobile military hospital.[4] A spokesperson of the Argentine Foreign Office commented: "...This is part of our bond with China, which is a solid relationship of mutual respect, and ties that go above and beyond our strong trade exchanges" (Reuters, 2020).

The U.S. for its part expressed interest in providing aid to the South American country, as an embassy official in Buenos Aires stated to Reuters toward mid-March: "This week we plan to make funds available to the Argentine authorities for combating the coronavirus", adding, "We are considering the possibility of additional donations" (Reuters, 2020). Towards mid-June, the aid provided by the U.S. to Argentina in the fight against the pandemic amounted to US$ 300,000, allocated to aid for refugees and host communities (US Aid, 2020).

On April 13, 2020, Argentine Foreign Minister Felipe Solá praised China upon the arrival of a large shipment of masks,

4. This, although the same had been donated in 2015 (and included in that of 2017), during the administration of President Mauricio Macri (Argentina.gob.ar, 2019).

gloves and protective suits. The boxes containing the health supplies were labeled with Chinese and Argentine flags and a quote in both languages from the Argentine poem by José Hernández, "Martín Fierro the Gaucho", in an allusion to the kinship between the two nations. "Let brothers be united, this is the first law; let them have true union, in whatever time" (Clarín, 2020). It was an original touch that nonetheless attracted criticism from certain sectors of the Argentine opposition. It was anticipated that China would send, in three separate consignments, 53,500 reagent kits; 405,000 thousand medical masks; 14,000 protective suits; 20 ventilators; 2,500 pairs of gloves; 2,000 pairs of goggles; 700 thermometers; 1,000 shoe covers, and two thermographic systems. The supplies would be delivered by the Chinese government itself, by the embassy in Argentina, by the city of Hangzhou, and by companies such as Alibaba, Huawei and Envision Energy. If the health situation in China remained under control there would be further donations, especially of ventilators (Observatorio Sino-Argentino, May 2020).

Through April, May and June, the health and medical cooperation to respond to the pandemic continued. According to Ambassador Guillermo Justo Chaves, Cabinet Chief of the Argentine Foreign Ministry, the cooperation was effected through the shipment of medical supplies and products, holding video conferences to share medical experience between various authorities and experts, and facilitation to enable Aerolíneas Argentinas to carry out an unprecedented airlift operation to Shanghai to pick up supplies and transport Argentine and Chinese citizens to Shanghai (Dangdai, 2020).

Also worthy of note is that, as of the 1st of June, there had been 17 special flights to Shanghai and 15 more planned for the remainder of June. The returning flights to Argentina carried reagents, detection tests, machines for fabricating masks, face shields, protection and isolation suits, ventilators, protective gloves, infrared thermometers, regular thermometers, masks, goggles, swabs for performing detection tests, magnetic stands, etc. All of the supplies were delivered to different destinations, at the national as well as the provincial level, including to specialized medical facilities. The supplies totaled 280 tons, plus another 10 tons of donations from Chinese entities[5] to their Argentine counterparts (Dangdai, 2020).

The government of the Province of Buenos Aires reported on June 5, 2020 that two ships had left Shanghai with 33 containers of supplies on board and would arrive on July 1. To give an idea of the magnitude of the medical supplies and products being shipped from China, the cargo on board equaled the air freight capacity of 15 cargo planes. Subsequently, the Argentine

5. Such as Envision Energy, Cofco International Argentina SA, Bank of China Argentina, China Communications Construction Company, Shenzhen Mammoth Foundation, and the BGI Group.

Defense Ministry reported the arrival of a shipment of medical supplies donated by the PRC for the protection of military health workers. The supplies included thermometer guns, raincoats, masks, gloves, goggles and smart helmets equipped with thermal sensors. The donated material arrived on the 24th special China flight of Aerolíneas Argentina and was received by Defense Minister Agustín Rossi. The Chinese donation reached Argentina in crates that also bore labels with the abovementioned verse from the book "Martín Fierro" (Infodefensa.com, June 2020).

Perspectives of the Post-Pandemic Bilateral Relationship

The U.S. and China are the two most important partners of the majority of Latin American countries. The U.S. economy is expected to contract by 5.9%, while the Chinese economy should grow by 1.2%. The latter is a precarious figure for Chinese economic levels; however, it is at any rate a positive platform for a reactivation in 2021. The subcontinent depends on the exploitation of its natural resources, which means that the governments' revenues are contingent on resource extraction. The wealth generated by the exploitation of non-renewables, i.e., oil, gas and minerals, accounts for between 3% and 7% of the subcontinent's GDP. A drop in the price of these products will have a considerable negative impact on the economic situation of the Latin American countries.

According to the figures of the Economic Commission for Latin America and the Caribbean (ECLAC), the subcontinent's GDP will register a contraction of -5.3%—its worst drop since the crisis of 1929. It is likewise forecasted that exports will fall by 15%. The combined scenarios of a trade slowdown, a drop in commodity prices, and strained lender-debtor relationships could compel some countries in the region to seek urgent economic assistance abroad (Caballero, 2020).

Despite the strong impact that Covid-19 will have on the Latin American economy, some quarters envision a recovery through trade with China. As stated by researcher Santiago Bustelo of the Argentina-China Study Center at the University of Buenos Aires (*Centro de Estudios Argentina-China,* ACSC; *Universidad de Buenos Aires,* UBA) in April this year, "despite the global economic and logistical standstill caused by Covid-19, there is room for optimism". He based his assertion on "the reestablishment of industrial activity in China and [the latter's] continual demand for the products that Latin America exports" (China Hoy, 2020).

The researcher added, referring specifically to Sino-Argentine trade, "[China]'s demand for the region's products will continue. In fact, exports to China from various Latin American countries can be observed to have risen in the first quarter of the year...as (in the case of) Argentine meat exports" (China Hoy, 2020).

This is evidenced by the figures from the Argentine Beef Promotion Institute (*Instituto de Promoción de Carne Vacuna de la Argentina,* IPCVA), indicating that between January and April 2020 China was the primary destination of Argentine beef exports. Said figures break down as follows: in January 2020, total sales to China amounted to US$ 141,127 (or 72.6% of total export volume); in February, US$ 79,326 (55%); in March, US$ 110,122 (66.7%), while total sales recorded in April reached US$ 160,767 (71.6%) (IPCVA, 2020).

Within a pre-pandemic context of an inward-turning U.S. economy, and the new reality of the impact of the Covid-19 crisis on supply chains, the pressing question then becomes: "What will be the future of the Chinese economy's linkage to the external sector?" The PRC should probably diversify its supply sources by replacing U.S. products with equivalent alternatives, besides developing other locally-manufactured products that will reduce its overseas dependence.

There is also the question of whether, as a result of the crisis, the government of the PRC will continue supporting the internationalization of Chinese capital with the same momentum as it has done thus far, or whether the Chinese state's financial clout will be redirected toward its domestic market. Researcher Robert Evan Ellis believes that Beijing will increase its presence on the subcontinent. In his opinion, Chinese companies would become "better positioned" thanks to the support they would receive from the Chinese government, as well as from their financial partners, "to expand their role in the global supply chains through the acquisition of strategic assets that are in bankruptcy or that local companies are looking to sell" (South China Morning Post, 2020).

Professor Mauricio Santoro of Rio de Janeiro State University (*Universidad del Estado de Río de Janeiro*), shares this opinion and considers that China's economic presence in Latin America will grow because the other major economic partners of the subcontinent (the U.S. and the E.U.) "are moving toward a huge recession...and Latin America is headed for an extremely serious economic crisis." Thus, "China could be the provider of much needed trade, investment and health aid" (South China Morning Post, 2020). The subcontinent could rise to its challenges if it had a more sophisticated agricultural sector. This became evident in 2019—at the height of the trade war between the U.S. and China—when Brazil increased its purchases of China's soybeans, thanks to the trade tariffs that the PRC levied on its rival (Caballero, 2020).

The Ecuadorian-Taiwanese academic Po Chun Lee takes his analysis farther, arguing that "China has the opportunity of the century in Latin America and the Caribbean, because most of the developed countries are planning divestments in their overseas operations and preparing to repatriate their supply chains". According to Lee, this situation would enable the PRC to continue expanding its overseas influence, as "one of the few countries able to offer the complete package"—financing, construction and maintenance of infrastructure projects (South China Morning Post, 2020).

Against this backdrop, Latin America should increase its sales of products with more value-added and support the private sector so that a new generation of enterprises (for example, food companies) can capitalize on Chinese niche markets. Thus the trade with China would also be successfully diversified. Regional value chains should be added on to this that meet strict quality standards, like those in force in the E.U. (Caballero, 2020). Likewise, the subcontinent needs to reduce gaps in its infrastructure and integrate borders to make use of trade corridors that connect it to the Asia Pacific markets. Latin America can then dovetail its needs with China's interest in developing and financing infrastructure works—which is the essence of the Belt and Road Initiative (Caballero, 2020).

Along with taking advantage of opportunities in traditional economic sectors, there are those who anticipate that there will be greater Chinese influence in such areas as technology and telecommunications. Jude Blanchette and Jonathan Hillman, researchers at the Center of Strategic and International Studies (CSIS) in Washington, D.C., believe that the pandemic "is already offering new opportunities" to China as a digital infrastructure provider. Thus, in their opinion, "the Digital Silk

Road will accelerate and expand" (South China Morning Post, 2020). However, this is one of the areas where the backlash from the U.S. is tremendous, as various governments in the region have experienced. Finally, Latin American needs to boost cooperation in other areas that enable the consolidation of the trade relationship; for example, more investments in the industrial sector. According to the above-referenced researcher Santiago Bustelo, in this way "the competitiveness and value added of the products exported by Latin America can be increased" (China Hoy, 2020).

On another front, the existence of over 40 Confucius Institutes on the subcontinent, of exchanges between thousands of students and teachers, and the visits to China by hundreds of Latin American journalists contribute to the building of bridges that facilitate mutual knowledge and understanding. The discourse of "cultural distance" between China and Latin America is fast losing relevance. Consequently, a sound substrate is in place, so that once the Covid-19 pandemic has passed, then political, economic, cultural and scientific-technological relations can advance toward a new era. It is a new era that can open a door for Latin America to a change in practices, norms and international institutions that can usher in a more just political and economic world order. It calls for an exercise in foreign policy that will know how to balance Latin American countries in the midst of the tensions between the U.S. and China. The

"Community of Shared Destiny for Humanity" (*Comunidad de Destino Compartido para la Humanidad*) that China proposes to build is a project for an integrated global system aimed at improving the international system. Its philosophical substrate is Chinese wisdom, and its material tool, The Belt and Road Initiative (*Una Franja, Un Camino*) (China Hoy, 2017).

The Case of Argentina: New Opportunities

For China to be Argentina's primary trading partner could be sustainable over time, given that the PRC has a greater capacity to finance Argentine exports than does Brazil. China offers tariff incentives of up to 75% on imports, depending on the category of merchandise (conditioned on official guarantees).

A major challenge are the possibilities for smaller-scale companies to export their products to China. In the words of the above-cited expert Emma Fontanet, there are opportunities in niche markets. However, associativity is required between the companies through the creation of export consortiums. As an example, the Fundación ICBC expert referred to the work of an exporter group of PyMEs (*Pequeñas y Medianas Empresas* or Small- and Medium-Sized Companies), wineries in the province of Salta that produce high-end wines for a select developing market. The five wineries share container and promotion costs. There are, besides, peanut-producing companies that have partnered based on the same modality (Bestani, 2020).

A business opportunity has arisen for Argentina to do business with China based on the levying of an 80.5% import tariff on Australian barley that effectively excludes it from the market for Chinese importers. Aside from this, the PRC would stop importing Australian wines. Furthermore, in mid-May China suspended the beef imports from four Australian establishments due to sanitation issues (Consejo Argentino-Chino, 2020), albeit also determined by the growing tensions between Australia and China.

Still another opportunity that has opened up for Argentina is the increased demand for Vitamin C among Chinese consumers as a result of the pandemic. On June 10, 2020, the formalities for the startup of exports of Argentine juices were completed after 20 years of intense negotiations. Citric, a company with home offices in Tucumán, in the center-north of Argentina, is set to begin exporting fruit juices to the PRC. The company anticipates that in the coming years it will export 5% of its total production, over half of which will go to China (Observatorio Sino-Argentino, 2020).

Likewise, despite the fact that pork sales have also been affected by the drop in prices, experiencing falls of up to 30%, the Chinese deficit in this sector due to swine flu is opening up another opportunity for increasing Argentina's exports. Based on a new memorandum with China the government, has plans for increasing pork exports, which totaled 1,000 tons last year (Observatorio Sino-Argentino 2020).

Still another opportunity on the horizon for Argentina would be to open up for commercial use the Aerolíneas Argentinas air route that is currently transporting medical supplies from China, and keep it operating for tourism after the pandemic has ended. There is government interest in implementing the waiver of tourist visas for Chinese nationals, which could break the country's tourism record of 70,000 visitors per year. Air connectivity would likewise be promoted through shared flight codes and leveraging the tourism flows between China and Oceania (Ng, 2020).

A measure in favor of all the above is the decision of the Fernández administration to open a new consulate in Chengdu, the capital of Szechuan Province, or in Chongqing, a municipality under the central government's direct administration (Ng, 2020).

Also open to Argentina is the option of taking advantage of the bi-oceanic corridors that offer direct access to the Pacific, through synergy with Chile and its free trade agreement with China. Even the more than 30 bilateral consultation mechanisms in place between Argentina and China, which have been underutilized in recent years, could be leveraged much more. An example is the *Comisión Binacional Permanente* (Permanent Bi-national Commission), which has not met for three years.

Final Reflections and Prospects

The U.N. General Assembly (*Asamblea General de las Naciones Unidas,* AGNU) adopted a resolution regarding Covid-19 on April 2, 2020 that called for "intensified" international cooperation to defeat the pandemic caused by the novel coronavirus (AGNU, 2020). It was the first resolution adopted by the General Assembly on the pandemic, and a very timely one because the pandemic is a threat to human health, safety and well-being that not only wreaks havoc on the populace, but continues to spread its contagion. The call for "intensified international cooperation" was (and will be) indispensable for containing, mitigating and defeating the pandemic, through the exchange of information, scientific knowledge and best practices, in observance of the World Health Organization's guidelines.

The benefits of an interconnected world should be taken advantage of to share information and knowledge on how to cope, not just with the health challenges, but with the environment, climate, food supply and education challenges as well. In this way, the eruption of crises such as the one triggered by Covid-19 can be avoided. In this sense, the reformulation of certain intergovernmental organizations is of central importance, as they should be the ideal ambit from which to materialize genuine cooperation between the states. Essentially, to reinforce the validity of multilateralism.

With its campaign for international cooperation, China for its part emerged as a key actor in the worldwide fight against the pandemic. This invites us to reflect on whether the pandemic, aside from being a humanitarian disaster, has also been a geopolitical crossroads. The crisis generated by Covid-19 has focused the world's attention on the political, economic and social models of the U.S. and China; hence it is natural that the question should arise as to how and when a transition to a new world order could occur, with China's decisive weight brought to bear in the ambit of international power.

Regarding Sino-Latin American relations, above and beyond the ongoing debate in certain media channels among journalists and academics as to whether the PRC is a "new colonizer" or a vital source of capital and technology, one thing is certain: Washington will not relinquish control over its "backyard" without a struggle. Consequently, pronouncements such as those of Mike Pompeo in 2018 and Kimberly Breier in 2019, or the content of the 2020 foreign policy statement, "U.S. Strategic Approach to the People's Republic of China", will continue to echo among us on the subcontinent.

Next year will be the centennial of the Chinese Communist Party, an occasion when the success and stability achieved in the economic, social and political spheres will be celebrated. While the PRC does not seek to replace the international order, the pandemic could well be the beginning of its recognition as a leading global protagonist. This conjuncture is offering China the strategic opportunity to transform practices and norms, that dynamize the international system.

As for Latin America, it finds itself before a strategic challenge of tremendous proportions, as a subcontinent located on a crossing of two roads: one is that of a hegemon, careless of its relations with its neighbors, and the other, that of a rising power.

IV. The Brazilian Experience of Combating Covid-19: Social and Economic Impacts

Marcos Cordeiro Pires [1]
Luís Antonio Paulino [2]

Abstract

This is a reflection on the Brazilian experience of fighting COVID-19 and its impacts on society and the economy. As the international statistics show, Brazil has become an epicenter of the pandemic, with over one million proven infections and over 50,000 deaths as of June 22, 2020. These figures reflect the inefficiency of the federal government's management of this problem, repeating many of the mistakes made in the U.S. Aside from the harm done to society, the pandemic is causing a recession in Brazil that is much worse than the world average forecasted by the IMF. This article develops the analysis of this situation in two sections: an Introduction and a brief Conclusion. The first section describes the response to the pandemic, underlining the disruptive actions of the President of the Republic and the role played by the cooperation between China and Brazil in minimizing its effects. The second section

1. Associate Professor - Universidad Estadual Paulista (Unesp). - Associate Professor Unesp.
2. Universidad Estadual Paulista (Unesp).

describes the social and economic impacts of the pandemic, demonstrating how the country is losing the battle against the virus and the recession.

Key Words: Brazil, COVID-19, combating the pandemic, social impacts, economic impacts.

1. Introduction

Consolidated figures as of June 22 indicate that Brazil was the leading country in South America in terms of the number of proven COVID-19 infections (1,111,348) and deaths caused by the pandemic (51,407). In absolute figures, Brazil is followed by Peru, Ecuador and Chile. However, in relative terms of deaths per million inhabitants Brazil's range of between 236 and 249 was not so disastrous, since despite the later arrival of the health crisis the U.S. had registered 370 cases per million, the U.K. 628 per million, Spain 606 per million, and Italy 573 per million. It is at any rate interesting to note that Colombia, Bolivia and Argentina recorded lower ranges (between 23 and 66 deaths per million inhabitants) than Brazil. However, the experiences of these Western countries was indicative of how far they lagged behind, in terms of capacity for coordination and efficiency, compared to such East Asian countries as China, with 3 deaths per million inhabitants, South Korea with 6, and Japan with 8.

Table 1 below illustrates this scenario.

Table 1. Countries with the highest incidences of COVID-19 in the world and in South America (By number of total cases, 22 June 2020)

#	Country. Other	Total Cases	Total Deaths	Tot Cases/ 1M pop	Deaths/ 1M pop	Total Tests	Tests/ 1M pop	Population
	WORLD TOP 10							
1	EUA	2.388.153	122.610	7.216	370	29.013.182	87.664	330.959.930
2	Brasil	1.111.348	51.407	5.229	242	2.430.347	11.436	212.525.202
3	Russia	592.28	8.206	4.059	56	17.289.691	118.477	145.933.256
4	India	440.45	14.015	319	10	6.950.493	5.038	1.379.678.183
5	UK	305.289	42.647	4.498	628	8.029.757	118.296	67.878.273
6	Espanha	293.584	28.324	6.279	606	5.162.909	110.426	46.754.429
7	Peru	257.447	8.223	7.811	249	1.517.930	46.054	32.959.833
8	Chile	246.963	4.502	12.922	236	982.353	51.399	19.112.361
9	Italia	238.72	34.657	3.948	573	5.013.342	82.915	60.463.455
10	Iran	207.525	9.742	2.472	116	1.449.420	17.262	83.965.446
	SOUTH AMERICA							
#	Country. Other	Total Cases	Total Deaths	Tot Cases/ 1M pop	Deaths/ 1M pop	Total Tests	Tests/ 1M pop	Population
1	Brazil	1.111.348	51.407	5.229	242	2.430.347	11.436	212.525.202
2	Peru	257.447	8.223	7.811	249	1.517.930	46.054	32.959.833
3	Chile	246.963	4.502	12.922	236	982.353	51.399	19.112.361
4	Colombia	71.183	2.31	1.399	45	620.288	12.194	50.869.620
5	Ecuador	50.64	4.223	2.871	239	139.333	7.901	17.635.866
6	Argentina	44.931	1.043	994	23	285.391	6.316	45.185.943
7	Bolivia	24.388	773	2.09	66	58.789	5.038	11.668.878
8	Venezuela	3.917	33	138	1	1.149.315	40.416	28.437.362
9	Guiana (FR)	2.458	8	8.236	27	8.061	27.011	298.43
10	Paraguay	1.392	13	195	2	57.895	8.12	7.130.320
11	Uruguay	882	25	254	7	57.687	16.608	3.473.480
12	Suriname	319	8	544	14	1.165	1.986	586.508
13	Guyana	205	12	261	15	2.147	2.73	786.470

Source: Wordmeters - COVID-19 Coronavirus Pandemic, 2020.

Brazil's figures are well above those of most of the South American countries, where policy coordination has been more efficient, as seen in the cases of Argentina and Uruguay. The planning level in Brazil for combating the health crisis should have been more sophisticated, but this was not the case. President Jair Bolsonaro chose not to lead the response to the pandemic, becoming instead a factor of sabotage for the various efforts to fight it, upon echoing conspiracy theories and news issuing from the U.S.

The result of this sabotage is that Brazil is currently experiencing the worst recession of its history, and at the same time is becoming one of the pandemic's epicenters, with over 1 million proven infections and more than 50,000 deaths.

2. The Brazilian experience in the fight against COVID-19

When the COVID-19 pandemic broke out in Brazil in March 2020, the country apparently had two advantages over the other countries. First, Brazil was aware of the pandemic's lethality and the national experiences in dealing with the disease such as those of China, Italy and Spain. Second, despite the funding problems of the health sector, Brazil has a Single Health System (*Sistema Único de Salud*, SUS) that guarantees the entire population of complete, universal and free access to health services (Ministerio de Salud, 2020). The Ministry of Health, state and municipal governments with their respective attributions are participating entities of the SUS. The Health Ministry is responsible for formulating general policies, while the state governments organize the more complex health services, and municipal governments make provision for the delivery of primary care services to families.

However, despite the central coordinating role that the federal government was duty bound to perform, President Jair Bolsonaro sabotaged all the initiatives for fighting the pandemic. Not only did the president deny the seriousness of the disease and advocate the use of inefficient medicines for its cure; he also showed contempt for, made light of and refused to support the policies of social distancing. He instead promoted large gatherings, rejected the use of protective masks in public places, and encouraged his supporters to boycott the initiatives fomented by governors and mayors to stop the spread of the coronavirus.

The Republic's institutions then attempted to contain Bolsonaro's tactics. The National Congress raised the health budgets to enable the states and municipalities to purchase mechanical ventilators, test kits and protective equipment for health professionals, as well as to enable protecting workers and companies from the economic impact of the quarantines. For example, while the Federal Executive advocated for a relief grant of R $ 200.00 (approximately US$ 40) for workers,

Congress raised this assistance to R $ 600.00 (nearly US$ 110) (Agencia Senado, 2020).

Likewise, on April 15, 2020, the Federal Supreme Court (*Supremo Tribunal Federal*, STF) ruled unanimously that the states and municipalities were invested with the autonomy to issue the order for social isolation. The ruling was a very important one for blocking the president's attempts to relax the quarantines. In his opinion, social isolation had to be restricted to persons at greater risk of contracting the disease, such as the elderly and those with chronic diseases.

But in spite of these measures, deficient coordination led to wastage of resources, lack of rationality, and several cases of corruption at the state and municipal level that are currently under investigation. As a result, Brazilian society did not respond adequately to the social distancing measures, which led to an exponential rise in the number of infections and made Brazil the second country in the world with the highest numbers of confirmed cases and deaths, behind the U.S.

2.1 The Evolution of COVID-19 in Brazil

The COVID-19 pandemic began to acquire importance in Brazil in early February 2020, when 34 Brazilians who were living in the pandemic's epicenter, Wuhan, China, were repatriated.[3] Around that time, information on how to deal with the disease also began to be disseminated in the media.

On the 26th of February, the first confirmed case of coronavirus in Brazil was identified: a 61-year-old man who returned to Brazil from Italy. Two days later, the Health Ministry launched a media campaign on open television, radio and Internet for the prevention of coronavirus contagion. The message to the population was to wash hands with soap and water, use 70% alcohol gel sanitizer, and refrain from sharing personal items. Up until then, 182 suspected cases were being monitored in 16 states.

On March 5, the first internal transmission of COVID-19 in Brazil was officially recorded. The other cases were linked to individuals who had visited Europe. The Health Ministry announced measures the following day for improving hospital services, reinforcing primary care, extending health facility hours, increasing the number of doctors, and providing telemedicine services (Ministerio de Salud, 2020).

On March 11, the World Health Organization (*Organización Mundial de la Salud*, OMS) announced that COVID-19 infections had become a pandemic and warned that the numbers of infected, deaths and of affected countries would be rising

3. The work carried out to describe the evolution of COVID-19 in Brazil was facilitated by the time line organized by the SANAR-MED (2020) portal, which highlighted some of the main events related to the pandemic. Aside from the information presented in the portal, other sources are especially cited.

in the following weeks. On the same day the Health Minister negotiated with the Legislative Branch for the release of up to R 5 billion for combating coronavirus in primary and hospital care facilities. The first COVID-19 death in Brazil occurred on March 12, though it was recorded by the Health Ministry three days later. The information was not rectified until June 27. The victim, aged 57, was a patient in a Sao Paulo hospital.

On March 16, Rio de Janeiro was the first state to enact a state of emergency to contain the epidemic. The measure would be quickly adopted by the rest of the states. It ordered the suspension of classes and all activities considered non-essential. However, these initiatives were insufficient because in areas with high rates of poverty and greater demographic concentration, social distancing turned out to be just around 30% instead of the recommendation of 60% and higher.

On March 20 Decree 6/2020, declaring a State of National Emergency, was passed by Congress effective until December 31 this year. The Health Ministry acknowledged that same day that community transmission of the virus was taking place throughout the national territory, although this type of transmission was not actually being observed in all the regions. At this time the federal government also defined by decree the essential services that could not be suspended: medical and social assistance, public safety, national defense, transport, telecommunications and Internet, water supply, sewage and garbage collection, electricity and gas supply, street lighting, delivery services, funeral services, radioactive substance control, health surveillance, pest prevention and control, postal services, environmental inspection, fuel supply and medical activities.

On March 27 Brazil joined the WHOs Solidary Study, coordinated by the Fundación Oswaldo Cruz (Fiocruz) and whose objective is to evaluate the effectiveness of four COVID-19 treatments.

On March 30, despite Jair Bolsonaro's boycott, the Northeast governors—most of whom belong to the opposition to the federal government—created a Scientific Committee which assisted in the public policy decision making for managing the pandemic. The Committee is coordinated by scientist Miguel Nicolelis and Sergio Rezende, physicist and former Minister of Science and Technology.

On April 8, the president advocated for the use of hydroxychloroquine as a cure for the disease and on the 16th of April Health Minister Luiz Henrique Mandetta was dismissed because of a difference of opinion with the president. He was replaced by Nelson Teich, an oncologist.

By May 3, 2020, Brazil had more than 100,000 COVID-19 cases and had recorded 7,000 deaths. Six days later the death toll had risen to 10,000. On May 13 Bolsonaro once again defended the use of chloroquine for treating coronavirus. Two days later the new Health Minister Nelson Teich tendered his resignation because he disagreed with the president's validation of the use of hydroxychloroquine. His post was taken over in the interim by General Eduardo Pazzuelo, who quickly signed a new protocol for the use of the drug. On May 31, Brazil had a total of 500,000 confirmed cases.

Given the negative impact of the pandemic on the country, the federal government tried to derail public opinion by suppressing the daily reports that it had been issuing on the pandemic. Between June 4 and June 8, the country did not receive updated official figures on the pandemic. Because of this, the major media outlets began compiling the current data from the states' health secretariats to keep the public informed. Days later, the STF forced the government to resume the daily publication of updated figures on the advance of the pandemic.

On June 19 the country passed the million mark of confirmed cases of infection. Three days later the death toll reached 50,617. Tables 2 and 3 show the evolution of the pandemic.

Table 2. Evolution of Number of Confirmed COVID-19 Cases

in Brazil (26 February - 22 June 2020)

Toltal de Casos Confirmados (26 fev - 22 jun)

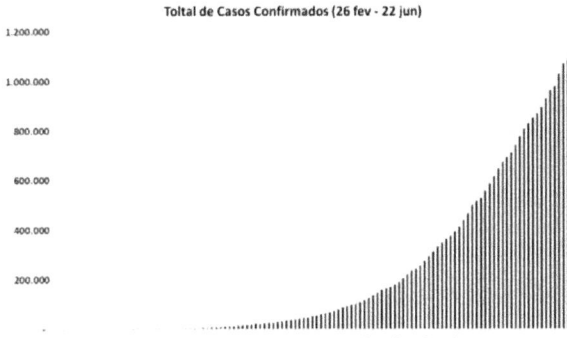

Source: Ministry of Health https://covid.saude.gov.br/

Table 3. Daily Evolution of Number of COVID-19 Deaths in Brazil (17 March - 22 June 2020)

Mortes por Dia (17 mar - 22 jun)

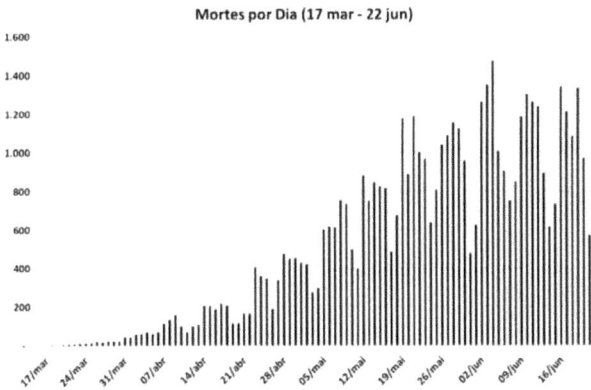

Source: Ministry of Health https://covid.saude.gov.br/

2.2 The Sabotage by Jair Bolsonaro

Jair Bolsonaro, like Donald Trump, reiteratively showed a dismissive, skeptical and arrogant attitude to the disease. He minimized its seriousness, expressing greater concern about the economic recession that was being triggered than interest in the health sector's initiatives. In the course of four months of crisis, he never showed a compassionate or empathic attitude toward his countrymen and women. On the contrary, he sought to boycott the preventive measures that the health ministers, state and municipal authorities were adopting.

The first time that Bolsonaro denied the seriousness of the pandemic was on March 10, when no deaths had as yet been recorded in the country, but the pandemic was already inflicting damage on Europe. According to [Bolsonaro]: "Much of what is out there is fantasy; the coronavirus issue is not all that the mainstream media are spreading. A part of the press successfully used the crisis to bring about the fall of oil prices." Then on March 16 he attempted to backtrack: "Alright, there is a problem for the elderly and for those with a [health] problem or disability. But it isn't all that they say it is." One day later he said, "Life goes on, no need to get hysterical. Just because a large group of people sporadically gather here or there doesn't mean that that's what has to be attacked." Moreover, on the 20th of March he compared COVID-19 to a "mild flu". "After the backstabbing I've endured, it'll take more than a mild flu to take me down."

In an open confrontation with the governors on March 28, mainly with Sao Paulo's João Dória, he declared: "I don't believe in this number [of deaths in Sao Paulo] ... [There's] a State there that took action on the basis of an order where finally, lacking a concrete cause of death, they fill in that it was corona virus".

On April 12, when the numbers of infected and deaths were rising faster, he denied the evidence, saying: "It seems the virus problem is starting to go away". Weeks later, on April 28, when asked about the fact that Brazil was now leading China in numbers of deaths, Bolsonaro disdainfully replied, "What of it? I'm sorry. What do you want me to do? I'm the Messiah but I don't make miracles". He was referring to his second name, Messias.

On June 11 he encouraged his supporters to invade the hospitals to try and embarrass the governors: "[If] there is a field hospital near you, a public hospital, find a way to go inside and film. Many people are doing it and more people need to do it, to show whether the beds are occupied or not. Whether the expenditures square up or not. That helps us", said the president.

On the 19th of June, the president once again criticized the policy of social isolation, mainly because of its economic consequences. "If it were up to me—but it's the Supreme Court (*Tribunal Federal*, STF) that says the governors are the ones who formulate this policy—I would never have [told the people] to stop going to work. And those aged 40 or younger are fine, the risk of [falling ill] is minimal".

In sum, President Jair Bolsonaro's posture regarding the national coordination effort to deal with the pandemic was extremely negative. Worth mentioning is the opinion expressed on June 23 by his former cabinet minister, Luis Henriquez Mandetta, regarding the president's performance:

"The President of the Republic clearly chose to give greater importance to the economic issue than to the health issue. He fell into a false dilemma, as though these things could be dealt with separately, when they are in fact interconnected.... This is a [crisis] of leadership that is shaking up other countries, because the world decided in favor of life first, and later for salvaging the economy. ...And he ended up the only world leader who has adopted [the former] line of action" (Revista Época, 2020).

In Mandetta's opinion, there is no longer a Ministry of Health. The former minister considers the Ministry as being under military control, and that the military follow none of the guidelines of the health authorities, abiding only by the opinions of the president.

2.3 Relations between Brazil and China in the midst of the COVID-19 Pandemic

The Bolsonaro government's lack of competency for responding to the COVID-19 pandemic was reflected in the relations between China and Brazil. Whereas the Chinese government tried to build bridges for cooperation through its embassy in Brasilia, the extreme right wing of the government took charge of echoing the prejudices expressed by President Donald Trump and his supporters, such as those of the president's son and of his education minister. Thus, before the cooperation between the two countries can be discussed, this problem that posed obstacles to the fight against the pandemic must be pointed out.

In March 2020, before the first COVID-19 case in Brazil was confirmed, many persons of Asian descent were the target of hostility in public areas. It is well known that the community of Japanese origin in Brazil is more numerous than the Chinese and Korean communities. Consequently, IBRACHINA, an NGO that works for cultural cooperation between Brazil and China, launched a media campaign against the aggressions. On the 18th of March, Congressman Eduardo Bolsonaro posted in his Twitter account, @BolsonaroSP, "Whoever has seen Chernobyl will understand what happened. Instead of the nuclear plant, think coronavirus; and instead of the Soviet dictatorship, think China, plus one time a dictatorship chose to conceal something dangerous and decadent rather than save innumerable lives. China is to blame and the solution would be freedom."

That same day Yang Wanming, Chinese ambassador to Brazil, answered, "Your words are an insult to China and the

Chinese people. This flagrantly anti-China attitude is inconsistent with your position as a member of the Federal Parliament and your role as an eminent public figure." As for the Brazilian foreign minister, on March 19 he posted on his Twitter account, @ernestofaraujo, "[T]he recent posts and the relationship between Brazil and China" demanding that Ambassador Yang Wanming apologize for his response to Eduardo Bolsonaro, for having allegedly offended the president of Brazil.

As of March 24, the diplomatic altercation seemed to have died down, thanks to Bolsonaro's telephone call to the Chinese president. Referring to the call the president tweeted from his @jairbolsonaro account, "During a telephone call this morning with the Chinese President Xi Jinping, we reaffirmed our bonds of friendship, information exchanges and actions concerning Covid-19, and the expansion of our trade ties".

On March 31, the Chinese Embassy released a letter declaring its willingness to help the country fight the corona virus. The letter was a reminder that China's measures against COVID-19 were effective and had been praised by the international bodies; it even went so far as to criticize the comments on social media against China for "inciting racism, xenophobia and even spreading hatred" (Consulado de China en Recife, 2020).

Meanwhile, on April 4, Minister of Education Abraham Weintraub created a new diplomatic crisis when he used Twitter to make a racist statement against China, employing characters from children's stories such as one with a speech impediment, mocking the pronunciation that some Chinese have when they speak Portuguese. Added to the tweet was an image of a panda bear and the Chinese flag.[4] The social media post caused the filing of a complaint against Weintraub for racism.

Independently of the friction created by the extreme right in the Brazilian government, while Luiz Henrique Mandetta was health minister contacts were initiated with the Chinese Embassy to seek the Chinese government's support to obtain medical equipment. Thus, on April 7, [Minister Mandetta] spoke with Ambassador Yang Wanming to coordinate actions against the pandemic. According to Mandetta, the conversation went as follows:

"The acquisitions in China had to be carried out in circumstances in which the market was extremely active and difficult. This afternoon I had a telephone conversation with the Chinese ambassador and we began working together with the vice minister in charge of business transactions, so that each purchase, each contract may guarantee the maximum transparency, soundness and information concerning the acquisitions" (Estado de Minas, 2020).

4. The work carried out to describe the evolution of COVID-19 in Brazil was facilitated by the time line organized by the SANAR-MED (2020) portal, which highlighted some of the main events related to the pandemic. Aside from the information presented in the portal, other sources are especially cited.

In view of the difficulties created by the federal government, a kind of "federative diplomacy" was implemented, through which the Brazilian states looked to China for the acquisition of health supplies (El País, 2020).

We illustrate this with the example of the actions of *Consorcio del Nordeste* (Northeast Consortium) which released a document in which it requests China's "support" and "collaboration" in the form of consignments of medical material, supplies and equipment. The governments of Distrito Federal, Pará, Santa Catarina and Sao Paulo, among others, have created their own direct channels to obtain the supplies they require. It is important to consider that a lack of coordination led to disparities in the prices of these goods of up to 400% (CNNBrasil, 2020). Moreover, as the newspaper *El País* mentioned, "The provocations aimed at China create a climate of apprehension in the middle of the pandemic and may harm Brazil's exports. The erosion of goodwill is felt when the time comes to close new accords with the Chinese," the association of exporters warned. "The governors are in a state of continual concern over the delivery of medical equipment for [fighting] corona virus" (El País, 2020a).

The abovementioned problems are illustrated by the events of April 3, when a consignment of 600 Chinese-made artificial ventilators purchased by the northeastern states was stopped at the Miami Airport, where the cargo was in transit for forwarding to Brazil. The vendor company canceled the contract for R $ 42 million (around US$ 9 million) that had been signed by the Bahía Government in representation of the region (Folha de São Paulo, 2020).

Another example of agreements between China and the state governments is a partnership between the State of Sao Paulo and the Chinese laboratory Sinovac for testing and production of a coronavirus vaccine (11 June). The vaccine is expected to be available in June 2021. The Instituto Butantan, a state-owned vaccine research center, will be the Brazilian counterpart of the Chinese laboratory (Folha de São Paulo, 2020a). In this context, there were various solidary initiatives organized by the Chinese government and by companies and civil society entities of Brazil's Chinese community. First of all, the translation of the book by Dr. Wenhong Zhang is worthy of mention. Entitled *Manual de prevención y control de Covid-19* (Manual for the Prevention and Control of Covid-19), its publication was sponsored by the Bank of China, *Oficina del Consejo de Promoción Comercial de China Internacional en Brasil* (Office of the China International Trade Promotion Council in Brazil), and by *Asociación Brasileña de Empresas Chinas* (Brazilian Association of Chinese Corporations). The work was coordinated by China Brasil and IEST Consultoría and was enabled by, among other institutions, *Instituto Confucio de la Unesp* (Confucius Institute of the State University of Sao Paulo,

UNESP).

Chinese companies in Brazil have been helping local communities. For example, on April 4 the telecommunications company Huawei made a donation to the government of Distrito Federal that consisted of 12,000 surgical masks and an AI system to assist in the diagnosis of Covid-19 (*Jornal de Brasilia*, 2020). On May 28, the Chinese company State Grid, which controls the power distributor CPFL, made a donation to the city of Campinas (SP) of 60,000 surgical masks for health professionals working in the municipal health network and treating patients with Covid-19. The Bank of China, through the China Consulate General, also made a donation to the city of Sao Paulo of 50,000 masks and 1,000 uniforms for treating patients diagnosed with corona virus (*Municipio de São Paulo*, 2020). Since the beginning of the pandemic in Brazil, IBRACHINA has been publishing "Observatorio Coronavirus" (Coronavirus Observatory), which provides information on the status of the virus in Brazil and in the world. As of the 27th of June, 146 reports had been published (IBRACHINA, 2020).

Clearly, the potential diplomatic problems created by the Brazilian government did not disrupt the cooperation between the two countries; however there can be no doubt that, had there been more political coordination, the harm caused by COVID-19 in Brazil would have been considerably lessened.

3. The Economic and Social Impacts of COVID-19 in

Brazil

At the start of the pandemic, the Economic Minister Paulo Guedes declared that Brazil would surprise with its 2% growth, in spite of the pandemic: "Brazil is not a leaf blowing in the wind, adrift on the international waves. Brazil has its own dynamic of growth," the minister stated on that occasion (Ribeiro, 2020).

The exact opposite happened. While most of the countries hardest hit by the pandemic began to resume normal activities, Brazil became the late epicenter of the coronavirus crisis and all predictions of its economic performance this year could not possibly be worse. President Bolsonaro's insistence on relaxing the social isolation in hopes of accelerating the resumption of economic activity was a failure. "The panorama is one of a very high number of cases and deaths from Covid-19, with a decline in economic activity in the second quarter" (Lamucci, 2020).

3.1 A fall in production with no prospects of recovery

The successive reviews of Brazil's 2020 GDP projections are increasingly pessimistic. The most optimistic forecasts which come from the government refer to a 4.7% decrease in the product. A report published by the U.N. on the world economic situation predicts that Brazil's GDP will fall by 5.2% this year

(Moreira, 2020). However, forecasts of a 6% to 7% decline are considered by many analysts as conservative. "A range of 7% to 10% would be closer to reality," say the economic consultants of a former president of the Brazil Central Bank (Conceição, 2020).

According to the Brazilian Institute of Geography and Statistics (IBGE), industrial production in March 2020 fell 9.1%, compared to February of the same year. This is the third biggest reduction in the country's history since the reports began to be issued in 2002, and below the most pessimistic estimates. "These figures reinforce the perception that the pandemic's effects on the country's economy may be worse than previously thought. This suggests that the first quarter performance was even weaker than forecasted" (Conceição e Villas Boas, 2020). The Brazilian Economic Institute of the Getúlio Vargas Foundation (*Instituto Brasileño de Economía,* IBRE; *Fundación Getúlio Vargas,* FGV) estimates a 12.9% decrease in Brazil's GDP for April with respect to the same month last year, the worst ever recorded for Brazilian economic activity in nearly 40 years (Villas Bôas & Saraiva, 2020). "With respect to March, services decreased by 11.7%, the retail market fell 16.8%, and industry 18.8%, all record-breaking figures in their respective historical series"(Valor, 2020).

A study done by IBRE/FGV affirms that the resumption of growth in Brazil will be slower than that of 90% of the countries, adding that, of the 192 countries studied, Brazil ranks

171st. In South America, only Venezuela's results will be worse than Brazil's. According to the study, "uncoordinated measures against the pandemic in [Brazil] will cause restrictions to remain in place longer, thus harming the economic recovery" (Gravas, 2020).

3.2 Inflation, Interest and Monetary Policy

The impact of the pandemic has caused a reduction of inflation and the probability is high that in 2020 inflation will fall below the level that was set by the Central Bank. The Central Bank's Focus Market Report published at the beginning of June forecasts an inflation rate for 2020 of 1.55% (Castro, 2020). The Central Bank's regimes of inflation targets predicts a variation of the Broad Consumer Price Index (IPCA) of 4% in 2020, 3.75% in 2021 and 3.5% in 2022, with a variability margin of 1.5 percentage points. According to IBGE, the IPCA suffered a deflation of 0.31% in April and 0.38% in May after rising 0.07% in March. "This is the biggest drop in prices since August 1998 (-0.51%) and the second largest in the historical series of the Index, which dates back to 1979. Considering just April, this is the biggest drop since 1980, the first year that provided monthly data" (Villas-Bôas, 2020).

The economy's weak performance has led the Central Bank of Brazil to successively reduce the basic interest rate (*Sistema*

Especial de Liquidação e Custodia, SELIC, the Brazilian federal funds rate). At its June meeting, the Central Bank's Monetary Policy Committee (*Comité de Política Monetaria*, COPOM) lowered the basic interest rate from 3% to 2.25% per year (Taiar & Ribeiro, 2020). Thus Brazil is nearing the point where monetary policy measures will no longer have an effect on reactivating the economy, leaving just fiscal policy, which the government is reluctant to employ and depends on the National Congress.

The government and the Central Bank have made resources available to keep the economy running. However, most of the money is concentrated in the banking system, which, given the risk of increased defaults, makes credit harder for businesses to access, especially if interest rates on loans to smaller businesses go up (Valor, 14/5).

3.3 Unemployment and fiscal policy

Since early 2019, when President Jair Bolsonaro took office, the government has been adopting a series of expenditure containment measures focused on reducing social welfare spending. Aside from reforming the social security system, which has much stricter rules for gaining access to benefits, especially for the poorest workers, deep budget cuts were made in all social areas (education, health and social assistance), as well as in infrastructure, science and technology. The result was a 1.1% growth in GDP in 2019 after four years of economic stagnation, during which time the Brazilian economy accumulated negative growth of around 5%.

The outbreak of the pandemic caught Brazil off-balance. Unemployment was at 11.6% in January 2020, equivalent to 11.9 million jobless, with 41.4% of workers or 38.8 million persons in the informal economy, for a total of over 50 million people in a situation of extreme vulnerability. The IBRE-FGV forecasts regarding the behavior of the unemployment rate indicate that it will rise to 18.7% by the end of 2020 and that, "unlike previous crises, this time the informal sector will no longer serve as a 'cushion' for those who have lost their jobs" (Villas-Boas, 2020).

Moreover, the government found itself forced by the circumstances and very reluctantly had to abandon its fiscal policy and adopt assistance measures for individuals and companies that have been hindered from working. The National Congress approved emergency assistance funds of R $ 600 (approximately US$110) during a period of three months for unemployed and self-employed persons who have lost their incomes due to the pandemic, as well as for individuals in extreme poverty who are beneficiaries of the program *Bolsa Familia* or Family Basket.

In just over two weeks, 50 million persons signed up to receive these emergency benefits. However, according to the president of the state bank in charge of disbursing the payments to these three large beneficiary groups, those registered in the Family Basket Program alone make up a base of 75 million people in the [records of] the *Ministerio de Ciudadanía* or the Ministry of Citizenship (Moreira, Furlan & Tauhata, 2020). This astonishing number of persons in a situation of vulnerability, much more than the impact of the pandemic, is revelatory of the tremendous precarity that most Brazilian workers are in.

Another red flag of how the poor are more exposed to the pandemic's effects were the findings of the National Household Survey (Continuous Pnad). The Study found that "the country had around 6 million households connected to the general water supply network who did not have daily access to water services. These households account for 11.5% of all households connected to the water distribution network in [their respective] localities" (Villas Bôas, 2020).

3.4 Foreign currency, foreign trade, direct foreign investment and balance of payments

Since end-January, foreign investors have been taking their money out of the poor countries. With the fall of world trade, low commodity prices and the disappearance of tourism, export earnings and the foreign currency they would otherwise supply are now in free fall. In Brazil, the devaluation of the real and the country's strong presence in the world markets of foodstuffs, such as grains and animal protein, contributed to a positive trade balance of US$ 6.7 trillion in April 2020. In fact, exports as well as imports diminished; however the drop in imports was more pronounced. The value of exports totaled US$ 18.3 billion but imports experienced a steeper reduction of 12.3%, totaling US$ 11.6 billion. Nevertheless, the final balance was the second highest result for the month in the historical series, exceeded only by that of April 2017.

Even in the middle of the pandemic, countries continue to purchase food. Exports to Asia rose 28.65% in April, and of these, exports to China grew by 29.5% despite the provocations from certain sectors of the government. An additional advantage of the connection to China was that the Asian country was emerging from its health crisis ahead of the other nations" (Valor, 5/12/2020).

A collateral effect of the crisis was Brazil's increased dependence on exports of basic products. According to IBRE/ FGV, "from January to April, commodities accounted for 67% of total exports" (Passarelli, 2020). It is the worst result of the last 20 years and shows that Brazil's de-industrialization, which was already deepening during the last two decades, is accelerating even more with the health crisis. In the current situation, the primary destinations of products manufactured in Brazil, such as Argentina and the U.S., are suffering from a general shutdown of activities. Conversely, China, the main destination of Brazilian products, is beginning to relax its social isolation measures, it is resuming economic activities, accelerating acquisitions of mineral and agricultural products to replenish inventories, and is anticipating new waves of Covid-19 contagion in other locations (Passarelli, 2020; Gottems, 2020). For these reasons, in May of 2020 China supplanted Brazil as Argentina's primary trading partner (Sá, 2020).

The current account, or the sum of trade and service balances, recorded a surplus in April of US$ 3.8 billion, leading some analysts to consider that the combination of an economic contraction and a depreciated exchange rate could eliminate the accumulated 12-month deficit at the end of this year (Osakake, 2020). If we consider that the current account deficit in 2019 was US$ 50.762 billion, this perspective could be considered positive; however, this is not the case.

The dollar's devaluation and the pandemic are forcing some companies to accelerate the nationalization of their production processes. La Mondial, a Brazilian manufacturer of household appliances, announced in April that it would be fabricating mixers, large fans for shops and churches, PA systems and heaters domestically, and in May added four more products to the list (Chiara, 2020). In response to the widespread lack of sanitizing gel, the paper container manufacturer Klabin developed a thickening material that is a substitute for Carbopol—an acrylic polymer used as a gel shaper and thickener—using raw materials derived from petroleum that transform liquid alcohol into alcohol gel. This product had been 100% imported from China and, in addition to its scarcity, a significant adjustment was made to its price. The new product is extracted from wood and was developed in just two weeks, thanks to a partnership between Klabin and the Senai Innovation Institute and the cosmetics manufacturer Apoteka, which produced the alcohol gel sanitizer in its factory located in Leme (SP) (Pereira, 2020).

Another secondary effect of the rise of the dollar with respect to the real was the Central Bank's positive cumulative result, thanks to the valuation of its international reserves. This amount varies according to the currency exchange rate and its impact on assets and liabilities in U.S. dollars.

Although a stronger dollar—whose appreciation is accumulating by over 45% with respect to the real this year—is provoking various positive effects on the economy as described above, it is also giving rise to problems. The rise of the dollar has raised R$ 907 billion, which Brazilian banks and companies will have to disburse to meet their foreign commitments. According to Central Bank data, the total debt of companies in Brazil is US$ 482 billion, equivalent today to R $ 2,846 trillion. This is substantially higher than Brazil's total currency reserves of US$ 343 billion. The Central Bank considers this particularly concerning for approximately 20% of the companies with no "exchange hedge" instruments to protect them against exchange rate variations. The data of *Fundación Instituto de Investigación Económica* (Economic Research Institute Foundation, FIPE) of the University of Sao Paulo indicate that, on average, large Brazilian companies with public and private capital currently maintain 57.7% of their debt in foreign currency (Jakitas & Holtoz, 2020).

Given this extremely worrying situation in Brazil's economy, the question naturally arises of what to do?

Fortunately, consensus is building in society among leaders and intellectuals of different persuasions that the anachronistic discourse of fiscal adjustment must be left behind in a time when the economy is in danger of definitive collapse from the lack of aggregate demand. Claudio Considera, Director of IBRE/FGV and a beacon of conservative economic thought in Brazil, says it best.

"That agenda has come to an end. We cannot insist on an adjustment for the pandemic; very soon we will have 17 million jobless. To avoid this we need to spend more on investment, public works, which have a great multiplier effect—construction employs 8.5% of formal labor. Either [the government] must convince itself of this, or the economy will not be reactivated in 2021" (Vasconcelos, 2020).

However, the administration's economic team is still

oblivious to this situation. They continue to advocate dogmas that are no longer taken seriously anywhere in the developed world, subject to assessments by risk agencies in a state of demoralization in their own countries. This is a major obstacle for Brazil to get out of the crisis. And its solution lies in the ground of politics.

4. Final Considerations

Clearly, the Brazilian experience of fighting COVID-19 has left much to be desired. The country is second in the world in number of infected and deaths and has yet to reach the peak of its pandemic. The federal government's failures have been many; i.e., it failed to recognize the pandemic's seriousness, it denied the scientific evidence, dismissed the successes in combating the pandemic, it did not coordinate the nation, and worst of all, boycotted the initiatives of governors and mayors who tried to apply internationally recognized good practices. In addition to the huge number of victims, the country is polarized and on the verge of an institutional breakdown. It is suffering from a huge waste of public resources because of inefficient public spending and corruption, and has been unable to maintain the two principal variables of risk: the lives of Brazilians, and economic performance.

Therefore, a positive aspect to consider is China's role

in backing the actions of Brazil, despite the diplomatic crisis created by certain authorities who replicated prejudices borrowed from the U.S. As we have seen, in the face of the federal government's lack of coordination, states and municipalities sought to articulate partnering with the Chinese government and companies in order to obtain resources needed for combating COVID-19.

Finally, the promises of 2% growth for this year that were announced by Minister Paulo Guedes proved to be demoralizing. The latest IMF report estimates that Brazil's GDP will have a fall of -9.1%, a performance well below the estimated world average of -4%. The country will emerge from the health crisis in a much worse condition than was imagined, with very high unemployment, hundreds of thousands of micro and small businesses in bankruptcy, and an explosion of public debt. And the prospects will be even worse if orthodox economic policies continue unchanged. These are indeed difficult times for the Brazilian people!

V. Why do People Refuse to Observe Social Distancing? Reflections on Covid-19 in the State of Amazonas, Brazil

Frederick Fagundes Alves, Lucas Vitor de Carvalho Sousa, Silvia Regina de Souza Rojas[1]

1. Introduction

In December 2019, a new type of pneumonia of unknown origin was first detected in the city of Wuhan, China. In late December, the Wuhan Municipal Health Commission issued an alert on the outbreak and a notification was sent to the World Health Organization (WHO). Prior to this, possible probable causes explaining the origin of the outbreak were ruled out, such as influenza, MERS and SARS. On January 7, 2020, it was discovered that a new, less lethal but highly transmissible new coronavirus was the origin of the disease (The Novel Coronavirus Pneumonia Emergency Response Epidemiology Team, 2020). The disease caused by the novel coronavirus was called COVID-19 and in just 30 days it spread from a single city to other provinces in China. The high speed of the disease's geographical spread and the sudden rise in the number of cases overburdened health services in China, mainly in Wuhan City

---

1. Department of Economics and Analysis, Universidad Federal de Amazonas.

and Hubei Province (Wu & McGoogan, 2020).

Given this situation, on January 23, 2020, the Chinese government adopted several measures to contain the transmission of the novel coronavirus, such as limiting the movement of people in and out of Wuhan and mobilizing all sectors of government to prevent the spread of COVID-19 (The Novel Coronavirus Pneumonia Emergency Response Epidemiology Team, 2020). Among the measures to contain the epidemic adopted by the Chinese government, was the construction of field hospitals in a few days with hundreds of beds, in an organized effort that amazed the world, and at the same time demonstrated that this was a problem demanding quick responses.

As was to be expected, global tourism and China's strong position in it and in international trade caused COVID-19 to quickly cross China's borders, and on March 11, 2020, the WHO recognized that this was not just an epidemic, but a COVID-19 pandemic that had hit virtually every continent. As China had done in the face of a new disease without a proven effective treatment and without a vaccine, the WHO recommended social distancing as a measure to reduce the spread and circulation of the novel coronavirus, SARS-Cov-2 (World Health Organization, 2020). However, contrary to what took place in China, a large part of the Brazilian population did not observe this recommendation (In Loco, 2020).

Given this noncompliance, the number of infected people rose more and more, especially in countries such as Brazil and the U.S., which have recently become the epicenters of the disease spread and contagion. The total number of cases of COVID-19 in Brazil exceeds 1.9 million people infected, and around 73,000 deaths towards mid-July. Amazonas, the Brazilian State with one of the highest rates of incidence and mortality of COVID-19, has 85,000 cases of COVID-19 and 3,048 deaths in total. China, an overpopulated country with 1.4 billion inhabitants, has 85,000 confirmed cases of COVID-19 and 4,641 deaths.

The rapid spread of the coronavirus in Amazonas led the state government decree, on March 23, 2020, of a state of public calamity as well as the implementation of social distancing measures. Public and private establishments were ordered to close and only essential services continued to operate. The purpose of this measure was to reduce the speed at which the virus was spreading so as not to overload the Health System.

In recent weeks, the number of cases of COVID-19 and deaths from it has increased, especially in Brazil as a whole. The situation has led to the idea that the social distancing recommended by the health authorities and constantly disseminated by the media as the primary preventative measure against COVID-19, has not been observed by much of the population.

Therefore, this study seeks to answer the following question: Why does a significant part of the population refuse to observe social distancing?

It presents data and describes the evolution of COVID-19 infection in Brazil and in the State of Amazonas, and it discusses why people tend not to follow the social distancing recommended by the health authorities. This discussion is relevant given the clash between the high rates of infection and death caused by COVID-19 on the one hand and, on the other, the reiterative pressure from public servants, companies and a sector of the population for restarting economic activities.[2]

2. The Pandemic Breaks Out in the State of Amazonas

According to Brazil (2008), the growth rate of a given population is the variation in the number of individuals found in a given geographical space during a given period.

The growth rate makes it possible to evaluate the performance of socioeconomic variables and the effects of decision-making. To this end, this work initially shows the evolution of COVID-19 infections and deaths in the state of Amazonas and Brazil and verifies the growth rate of these variables over the weeks. Moreover, the study seeks to compare the spread of the pandemic between Amazonas and the rest of

2. All figures recorded as of July 14, 2020.

the country.

This was done based on the period from March 13 to June 25, 2020, both for the State of Amazonas and for Brazil. This period is justified based on the first case diagnosed with COVID-19 in Amazonia, on March 13. In addition, these days will be subdivided into fifteen weeks to make a comparison of growth rates of the number of people infected and the deaths over these weeks. Therefore, the first week covers the days from 13/03 to 19/03 and the fifteenth week covers 19/06 to 25/06. The data used for this study was obtained from the Secretariat of Health of the State of Amazonas (Susam, 2020) and from the Ministry of Health (Brazil, 2020).

On March 11, before the first confirmed case of corona virus in the State of Amazonas, the World Health Organization (WHO) substituted the term "epidemic" for "pandemic" on the assumption that the disease was already on all the continents.

In the first week that was analyzed, more precisely on March 17, the first death from COVID-19 in Brazil was recorded, while the first death in Amazonas occurred the following week, on March 24, one day after the publication of the first state decree recommending social distancing in the state of Amazonas (23rd of March).

Several economic activities considered non-essential had to be temporarily closed down in observance of the social distancing recommended by national and world health authorities. As a result, the unemployment rate rose to 12.9% during the trimester of March to May, reaching 12.7 million people,[3] and millions have lost some or all of their income. To provide financial assistance to these people, the federal government announced the enactment on April 2 of Law 13.982/2020 that provides social benefit money transfers in the amount of R$ 600. In the midst of the pandemic and as the cases of infection and deaths rose, people started to form long lines in front of the offices of the Federal Economic Fund (*Caixa Econômica Federal*) and lottery houses to sign up for the Individual Registration List (*Registro de Personas Físicas*, CPF), get their data corrected and obtain information on the registration application of individuals eligible to receive emergency assistance (April 9, Week 4). In this time period, as Table 1 shows, in Brazil there were 47 cases of COVID-19 per million inhabitants per week, while in Amazonas there were approximately 165 cases per million inhabitants. On April 17, the sixth week of the reporting period, the federal government did not agree with the social distancing guidelines proposed by the Ministry of Health and decided to replace the then-Minister of Health, Luiz Henrique Mandetta, with Nelson Teich. As of that date Brazil already had 33,682 infected persons and 2,143 deaths from COVID-19. In the State of Amazonas there were 1,809 infected persons and 145 deaths

3. Source: https://g1.globo.com/economia/noticia/2020/06/30/desemprego-sobe-para-129per- cent-em-maio.ghtml

from COVID-19.

Less than a month after the change of ministers, Nelson Teich was already at odds with the federal government, which was pressuring him to augment the list of authorized economic activities during the pandemic and relax social distancing. On May 15, he tendered his resignation as Minister of Health.

By Week 10 of the period under analysis, Brazil had accumulated 218,223 cases of COVID-19 and 14,817 deaths, and the week following, or Week 11, the State of Amazonas reached its highest number of infections—2,652 cases per million inhabitants. However, it appears that Brazil, has not yet reached its peak of cases, as seen in Table 1. In the final week of the analysis (Week 15), Brazil had approximately 1,189 cases of infected persons per million inhabitants.

In contrast to the disorganization in Brazil's observance of the pandemic response guidelines, in just 12 days China built two temporary hospitals with capacity for treating 2,600 patients, and sent hundreds of doctors from different parts of the country to Wuhan. As one method of preventing the spread of the virus, the Chinese government has restricted travel between cities and imposed limits on entry to and exit from Wuhan. Additionally, police authorities used drones equipped with loudspeakers to control citizens' use of masks and health workers did door-to-door readings of residents' temperature.

Table 1: Total cases of COVID-19 per million inhabitants and weekly growth rate in Brazil and Amazonas

| | Brasil | | Amazonas | |
	Casos	Tasa de Crecimiento	Casos	Tasa de Crecimiento
Semana 1	2.59	-	0.74	-
Semana 2	10.92	321.7%	15.75	2033.3%
Semana 3	23.77	117.7%	39.87	153.1%
Semana 4	47.33	99.1%	164.88	313.6%
Semana 5	59.81	26.3%	201.54	22.2%
Semana 6	90.73	51.7%	287.67	42.7%
Semana 7	170.78	88.2%	582.24	102.4%
Semana 8	236.62	38.6%	1192.29	104.8%
Semana 9	322.69	36.4%	1742.78	46.2%
Semana 10	509.97	58.0%	2014.46	15.6%
Semana 11	609.82	19.6%	2652.56	31.7%
Semana 12	840.85	37.9%	2541.33	-4.2%
Semana 13	894.07	6.3%	1849.59	-27.2%
Semana 14	834.24	-6.7%	1660.34	-10.2%
Semana 15	1189.51	42.6%	1607.19	-3.2%

Source: Prepared by the authors based on research data.

In Brazil and particularly in the Amazon, the slowness in adopting drastic measures in response to the pandemic has resulted in alarming figures. The number of victims affected by the virus in Amazonas is very high, especially when weekly numbers per million inhabitants are compared to Brazil figures as a whole. The population of the State of Amazonas is just 2% of Brazil's total population and in Week 9 Amazonas recorded five times more cases than Brazil. The total number of COVID-19 cases in the State of Amazonas already approaches the total cases in all of China.

While the total weekly figures of infected per million inhabitants in Amazonas is still higher than in Brazil, the number of infected in the State of Amazonas seems to be decreasing as the weeks pass. At the same time, in Brazil the total number of persons infected with COVID-19 is still trending upward.

Starting on Week 12, the total cumulative weekly cases per million inhabitants in Amazonas was lower compared to the previous week. The growth rate of total cases then started to decline to negative figures. Conversely, in Brazil only Week 14 recorded lower figures compared to the preceding week.

As for the number of fatalities, Table 2 shows that in Week 9 the State of Amazonas recorded 105 deaths per million inhabitants, while the weeks that recorded the largest number of deaths per million inhabitants in Brazil were Weeks 12 (34.58) and 15 (34.37). The total number of deaths per week in the State of Amazonas was also trending downward and as of Week 13, the number of deaths per million people in Amazonas was lower than that of Brazil.

Table 2. Total deaths due to COVID-19 per million inhabitants and weekly growth rate in Brazil and the State of Amazonas.

	Brasil		Amazonas	
	Fallecidos	Tasa de Crecimiento	Fallecidos	Tasa de Crecimiento
Semana 1	0.03	-	0.00	-
Semana 2	0.34	1083.3%	0.25	-
Semana 3	1.06	212.7%	1.23	400.0%
Semana 4	3.06	189.2%	8.37	580.0%
Semana 5	4.68	53.1%	20.92	150.0%
Semana 6	6.61	41.3%	27.32	30.6%
Semana 7	12.32	86.3%	47.00	72.1%
Semana 8	15.44	25.4%	93.76	99.5%
Semana 9	23.06	49.4%	105.57	12.6%
Semana 10	28.81	24.9%	94.74	-10.3%
Semana 11	31.92	10.8%	84.65	-10.6%
Semana 12	34.58	8.3%	47.74	-43.6%
Semana 13	32.82	-5.1%	21.16	-55.7%
Semana 14	32.50	-1.0%	16.73	-20.9%
Semana 15	34.37	5.8%	9.84	-41.2%

Source: Prepared by the authors based on research data.

At this time the State of Amazonas is recording around 2.46 deaths per million inhabitants per day, while Brazil as a whole is tallying around 5.43 deaths per million inhabitants per day.

This mortality rate per million inhabitants in Brazil is equal to 220% more deaths, compared to the current figure for the State of Amazonas.

Images 1 and 2 compare the number of infected and fatalities per million inhabitants from COVID-19 in the State of Amazonas and Brazil, using moving averages[4] with a weekly analysis interval. Image 1 shows that the number of people infected with COVID-19 in Amazonia is much higher than in

4. Moving averages are often used to analyze information over a certain period to smooth out short fluctuations and highlight long-term trends.

all of Brazil, when these values are standardized per million inhabitants. However, Amazonas already reached the peak of infections on May 29, while in Brazil the number of infected has still not flattened and continues to rise.

Image No. 1. Mobile average of numbers of infected with COVID-19 per million inhabitants in Brazil and Amazonas

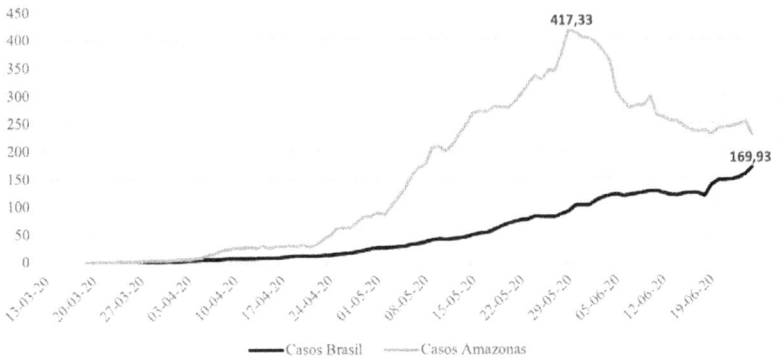

Source: Prepared by the authors based on research data.

Image No. 2 shows that the number of deaths per million inhabitants in the State of Amazonas is higher than that of Brazil, while the State of Amazonas registered, on average, around 16 deaths per million inhabitants on May 9; on the same day Brazil recorded on average 2.65 deaths per million inhabitants.

Image No. 2. Moving average of fatalities from COVID-19 per million inhabitants in Brazil and the State of Amazonas

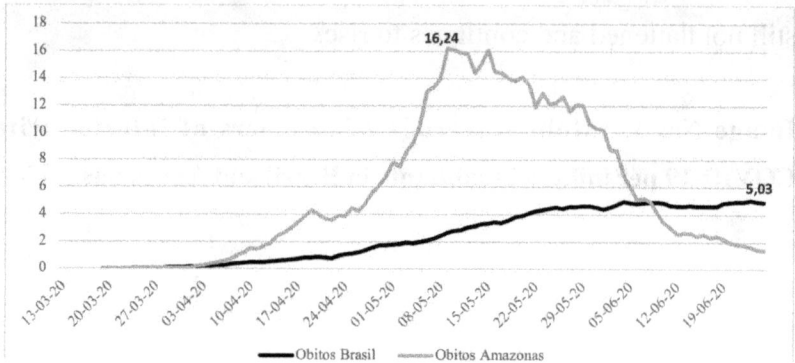

Source: Prepared by the authors based on research data.

From June 6 on, the number of deaths per million inhabitants in the State of Amazonas was lower than the same figure for Brazil.

At present Amazonia is recording an average of 1.4 deaths per million inhabitants, while in Brazil this figure is 3.5 times higher (4.91 deaths per million inhabitants).

These results show that even after over 100 days of the pandemic, the number of people infected in Brazil continues to rise and is showing no signs of falling, as has occurred in the State of Amazonas and in other countries. This could have to do with the low compliance with social distancing recommendations. In this respect, the following section discusses the social distancing recommendation and puts forward possible hypotheses for the non-compliance.

3. Social Distancing and Non-Adherence to this Recommendation

In the current pandemic scenario, one of the main recommendations for prevention of the COVID-19 disease is social distancing, since there are as yet no vaccines or drugs that are effective against the virus. Social distancing is a situation in which individuals stay home, go out as little as possible and have direct contact only with people living in the same household. This decreases the number of interactions between individuals and therefore the speed of virus transmission. The pressure is then lessened on hospital services, which could not cover the treatment and care requirements of infected persons without mandatory distancing (WHO, 2020). This recommendation is also widely publicized in the media.

According to the study by Almeida et al. (2020), on the epidemiological curve of COVID-19 in Manaus, the capital of the State of Amazonas, the number of new people infected will go down rapidly with a degree of social distancing greater than 60%. In other words, a maximum of 40% of the population is expected to leave their homes, thus social distancing will stay at 60%. However, according to data from *Mapa Brasileño de COVID-19* (MBC, 2020), in just one day, Sunday, April 19,

2020, there was 60% distancing in Amazonas. The question then is, despite the recommendation to observe social distancing, given its wide dissemination in the media, even of the resulting chaotic scenes in many hospitals, why does a significant part of the population refuse to observe social distancing? There is not a ready answer, but some hypotheses can be put forward.

a) The inertia of the status quo: People don't like change and prefer to act as they have always done. With respect to public policy, decision makers are usually averse to change as well and this can have negative consequences in emergency situations where atypical decisions are necessary (Howlett, 2012; 2014). In Brazil, pre-pandemic economic policy was based on actions oriented toward long-term growth, job creation, interest rate cuts and controlled inflation (*Plan gubernamental propuesto*, 2018). In other words, such was the status quo of economic policy in Brazil. However, with the advent of the pandemic and growing numbers of infected and fatalities in the country, many mayors and governors have enacted social distancing measures. But these decrees do not converge with the President's discourse and personal attitudes. He considers that a dilemma exists between economic growth and social distancing, and given these two alternatives he opted for the first one—maintaining the status quo. This position leads us to believe that the President is extremely reluctant to take on the risk of jeopardizing economic progress despite all the recommendations to the effect that it is what must be done to confront the pandemic.[5] Said aversion may lead governments to adopt procedures and strategies that will minimize a problem and deny the need for substantive measures to respond to it, instead of taking positive steps toward a solution (Howlett, 2012; 2014). These strategies include trying to reduce the problem's importance and reach, exercising gradualism or questioning the legitimacy and credibility of those who advocate adopting more substantive actions (Saward, 1992).

b) Fake News: People tend to believe the news that their families and friends share with them; they are not in the habit of confirming the veracity of the facts. People often believe such news more than the mainstream media, for example the recent case of empty coffins that led the people to believe that the number of COVID-19 deaths in the State of Amazonas was being manipulated.[6] According to Bayer et al. (2019), fake

5. It must be emphasized that, from an economic point of view, there is no dilemma between economic growth and the preservation of lives (through social distancing). However, given the President's speech in which he stated that social distancing was a "medicine" that could "kill" the economy, this means that for him there is a dilemma. Of course, the President's real dilemma may be the political cost of the pandemic and the face-to-face elections in 2022; however, this issue lies beyond the scope of this Technical Note. Source: https://noticias.uol.com.br/comprova/ ultimas-noticias/2020/05/04/foto-de-caixao-vazio-e-usada-para-enganar-sobre-mortes-por-co-vid- 19-no-am.htm

6. Source: https://noticias.uol.com.br/comprova/ultimas-noticias/2020/05/04/foto-de-caixao-va- zio-e-usada-para-enganar-sobre-mortes-por -covid-19-no-am.htm

news is technically disinformation or "propaganda" meant to disseminate false content that is published to produce a political effect in a matter of public interest. The cited study also states that disinformation can come from governmental or non-governmental, domestic or foreign agents. The elements of disinformation and propaganda (i) are designed to be wholly or partially false, manipulative or deceptive, or they use unethical persuasive techniques; (ii) they address a matter of public concern; (iii) they are intended to create insecurity, hostility or polarization, or attempts to disrupt democratic processes; and (iv) they are disseminated and/or magnified with automated and aggressive techniques such as social bots, AI, etc., often used to make the "news" more visible to the public.

c) The discourse and opinions of decision makers: The discourse of decision-makers, above all those able to reach thousands or millions of people, can influence behavior. In the specific scenario of a pandemic, the attitudes and opinions of the political leadership can significantly affect individual health and the health services. Ajzenman, Cavalcanti and Mata (2020) sought answers to how the behavior of people in Brazil is affected by the words and actions of the political leader. Their findings reveal that after the president of Brazil publicly minimized the risks associated with the COVID-19 pandemic and advised against social distancing, the observance of social distancing in pro-government regions has lessened compared to the regions where there is less support for the government. In other words, presidential discourse affects people's behavior, especially in the municipalities where the president received the majority vote in the 2018 elections. Ribeiro and Ferrini's essay (2020) yielded a similar finding. In the municipalities of the State of São Paulo, where there are more than 300 thousand voters, the authors estimated the correlation between the percentage of votes for Bolsonaro in the first round of elections and how much social distancing was observed following the presidential speech of March 24, 2020.[7] They found a strong negative correlation (i.e., the higher the number of votes Bolsonaro got, the less people observed social distancing). In the same vein, an opinion poll conducted by Datafolha (2020) found that in the regions of Brazil where Bolsonaro is more popular, support for social distancing is lower than in regions where the President is less popular.

d) The Unidentified Individual Bias (or the Identifiable Victim Effect): Without a doubt, death is something that people are extremely averse to.

However, despite the more than 73,000 fatalities documented in Brazil because of COVID-19, many people began or continue

7. In the declaration of national income of March 24, 2020, the President advocated for relaxing social distancing.

to disregard social distancing. This may be due to the bias of the unidentified individual. It is a term attributed to the American economist Thomas Schelling, when he described how harm to a specific individual causes feelings of anxiety, guilt, reverence and responsibility. However, most of such feelings vanish when people are merely being informed of mortality statistics (Schelling, 1968). Brazil presently has over 210 million inhabitants, and although over 73,000 people died of COVID-19, the vast majority of the population is unaware of them. Although people may feel some degree of shock, the unidentified individual bias means that people do not change their behavior.

e) The Paradox of Social Isolation: The more people socially distance, the less contagion there is and people then tend to think that social distancing is unnecessary. Conversely, even with distancing there are cases of transmission, because not everyone is isolated. People who work in essential services such as health, safety and food production continue to work, which can cause viral transmission to them. This causes other people to believe that social distancing does not work. But, of course, if all people were not isolated, the number of confirmed cases of COVID-19 would increase more rapidly, which would lead to the collapse of health services. COVID-19 is a challenge for health systems as there is a lack of perception on the part of the general population that increased contagion affects the health system's response capability.

f) Socioeconomic Conditions: The Brazilians' socioeconomic situation was already a cause for concern even before the start of the COVID-19 pandemic. There were nearly 12 million jobless and 40.7% of workers were in the informal economy.[8] After the WHO confirmed the existence of a pandemic and once the virus was propagated to Brazil, the majority of the informal sector workers lost practically all their earnings and, at first, no government counterpart revenues were forthcoming. Even after the emergency benefit was approved of R $ 600 per person for a period of three months, the monthly payments are taking time to reach the people which causes them to jettison social distancing and look for some way to earn their livelihood instead.

All of these assumptions directly or indirectly influence people's decision to adhere or not to adhere to social distancing. Changing the status quo requires much discussion and awareness, especially when the decision-maker is strongly averse to change. Speaking of the president of Brazil, aside from his clear preference for the status quo, he shows signs of

8. Source: https://g1.globo.com/economia/noticia/2020/02/28/desemprego-fica-em-112percent- em-janeiro-e-atinge-119-milhoes-diz-ibge.ghtml
https://www.correiobraziliense.com.br/app/noticia/economia/2020/02/28/internas_economia,831073/trabalho-informal-cai-em-janeiro-com-aumento-de-trabalhador-com-cnpj.shtml

confirmation bias. It is a kind of cognitive bias that causes an individual to tend to remember, interpret, or research information that will confirm his or her base belief or hypothesis.[9] Their resistance to change is then reinforced. To the extent that the President minimizes the pandemic, the mayors and governors will be called upon to continue addressing the problem. Fake news pose a challenge for policymakers because they can shape people's behavior in accordance with a desired objective, often one that is detrimental to society. In this scenario of a pandemic, the spread of fake content becomes even more worrisome as it can lead to the discrediting of the health authorities, resulting in exacerbated transmission of the virus. Therefore, fake news must be fought with exemplary punishment for creators and propagators. The bias of the unidentified individual and the paradox of social distancing can be mitigated with awareness and quality information. Even the media have already shown the faces of COVID-19 victims and emphasized the importance of social distancing. Regarding the population's socioeconomic conditions, the federal government is responsible for accelerating the process of awarding and disbursing to the workers who have been affected by the social distancing, and thus prevent people from leaving their homes in search of an income.

9. The president of Brazil recently misrepresented the message of the speech delivered by the director general of the WHO, to imply incorrectly that the organization was aligned with his administration. Source: https://www.nexojornal.com.br/expresso/2020/03/31/Como-Bolsonaro-distorce-a-fala-do-diretor-geral-da-OMS

All of these possible solutions can take time before they are rolled out.

Since not just the State of the Amazonas but Brazil as well are both facing an emergency, the right way to maintain social distancing will be to create incentives. One of the basic principles of economics is that people respond to incentives. According to Mankiw (2016), an incentive is something that causes the individual to act due to the prospect of a reward or a punishment. From the perspective of public policy, the decision-maker can adopt a policy that will change the individual's cost-benefit position and thus cause them to change their behavior. The decision-maker shall then implement inspections and impose fines on those who do not observe social distancing, as is already the case in the European countries.

4. Conclusions: Looking to China

The purpose of this study was to analyze the evolution of COVID-19 in Brazil and in the State of Amazonas, and put forward hypotheses that will justify the failure to fully observe social distancing. Brazil is considered one of the epicenters of the COVID-19 pandemic, and of all the country's federal units, the State of Amazonas has been one of the most hard hit. The death toll of COVID-19 rose very rapidly and also affected the internment capacity of the cemeteries in the latter State.

COVID-19 is a new disease without a specific, scientifically proven and effective treatment or a vaccine, and therefore the primary recommendation of the medical authorities as a preventive measure is social distancing. When this measure is observed, it reduces the number of interactions between people and infections and, therefore, relieves the pressure on the treatment capacity of hospital centers. The measure was successfully adopted in China and resulted in a total number of cases and deaths that was much lower than that recorded in Brazil.

Despite the recommendation of social distancing, China's example as well as government measures such as the suspension of nonessential activities to bring about more distancing, the number of cases and deaths rose significantly in Brazil and in the State of Amazonas.

This outcome creates the false impression that social distancing does not work. In reality, however, what happened was that the population only partially adhered to social distancing and a certain polarization arose with respect to the acceptance and practice of the requested standards of care despite the wide media coverage and the decrees issued by municipal and state administrators. This led to the questioning of the possible reasons why social distancing did not receive strong support. The hypotheses put forward touched on the issues of maintaining the status quo, the dissemination of fake news through the social networks, the lack of alignment between the various discourses and opinions of decision makers, the bias of the unidentified individual in which the statistics do not stimulate personal identification, how the paradox of social isolation generates the feeling that implementing the requested isolation and health measures are not so necessary, and the Brazilian socioeconomic problem that generates insecurity, fear and the compelling search for daily sustenance.

Most of the solutions intended to justify the non-compliance with social distancing recommendations require time before they can be fully materialized, and in a pandemic situation it is essential for these measures to have an impact in the short-term so as to minimize disease transmission. Thus, given the pandemic's exceptional nature, exceptional measures must also be adopted. This was done in China in front of a critical emergency situation. In this context, the application of a fine for non-compliance with social distancing is worth considering as a short-term measure; although the issue requires a variety of socioeconomic solutions.

VI. Central America and El Salvador in Times of COVID-19:
Expected Impacts and Public Policy Proposals

Oscar Ovidio Cabrera Melgar[1]

Abstract

In this investigation we delved into the transmission channels of the shock to El Salvador's economy originated by the COVID-19 pandemic and the impacts expected on the population's living conditions and on aggregate supply and demand.

The effectiveness of the epidemiological policy is examined and the 85-day period of total confinement that was imposed that failed to flatten the infection curve. In the context of a rising infection rate, the scaling back of quarantine began and the return to formal economic activity, excluding the 70% employed in the informal sector.

The impacts of the pandemic have been translated as the more than 600,000 people who have fallen into poverty from the perspective of income, and a loss of at least 240,000 jobs. In

1. Óscar Ovidio Cabrera Melgar is the President of the Central American Development Foundation (Fundación para el Desarrollo de Centroamérica, FUDECEN) and former chairman of the Central Reserve Bank of El Salvador (Banco Central de Reserva de El Salvador) from June 2014 to May 2019.

2020, growth will decline by -7.2% and recover slightly in 2021 by 3.0%.

Faced by financial instability in the dollarized economy occasioned by the external shock during 2020 which has produced a current account deficit, policy makers decided to implement a policy of increased spending in response to the decline in tax revenues. Consequently, bonds were issued to cover the deficit, which increased the interest rate and exacerbated the fiscal deficit.

The evolution of cases in the Central American region is still in the accelerated propagation phase in Guatemala, Costa Rica and Honduras, while in El Salvador, Panama, the Dominican Republic and Belize, the number of recovered cases exceeds the active cases.

China has shared her tactics and achievements in the fight against the virus with the Central American countries with whom she maintains diplomatic relations, stressing an open, transparent and responsible approach to the dissemination of information, the sharing experiences of control and treatment of infected cases, and the provision of medical supplies for COVID-19 treatment.

The International Environment

The State Council Information Office of the People's

Republic of China (2020) published a white paper on the fight against COVID-19. "China in Action" summarizes the country's efforts to fight the pandemic from the first moment that the virus appeared and presents a time line of daily actions that were put in place since the emergence of the virus until the attenuation of the infection curve.

On January 30, 2020, the COVID-19 epidemic was declared a Public Health Emergency of International Concern by the World Health Organization (WHO) (Organización Panaméricana de la Salud, 2020). The epidemic's characterization as a pandemic meant that it had spread to several countries, continents or the entire world and was affecting large numbers of people.

The rapid measures of confinement adopted by the Chinese government enabled the containment of the virus' spread within one month. During the next two months, approximately, the number of active coronavirus cases were reduced to a single digit, and in around three months the infection curve was attenuated.

According to the white paper statistics, China's confirmed cases peaked on February 12, 2020 at 15,152, while on May 31, 2020, a total cumulative figure of 83,017 confirmed cases was confirmed. Of these, 78,307 infected persons had recovered and been released from hospital and 4,634 had died. The recovery rate was 94.3% and the mortality rate, 5.6% (Page 5). With respect to global statistics of the coronavirus outbreak as of

June 17, 2020, there were around 8.2 million people infected, of whom four million had recovered and over 443,000 had died. The Americas are in the phase of a gradual increase of cases as measured by the number of cases with a basic reproductive number from 0.9 to 1.5. The U.S. and Brazil stand out with the highest numbers of infected on the continent. The viral infection curve has been in remission in China and Europe while continuing to expand in the rest of the world.

Table 1. Number of COVID-19 Cases: Infected, Deaths and Recovered

	Infectados	Muertos	Curados
Mundo	8,176,651	443,765	3,956,537
Europa	2,410,127	18,886	1,290,045
América	3,978,032	188,746	1,630,332
EE UU	2,137,731	116,963	583,503
Asia	1,293,201	38,950	826,296
China	84,422	4,638	79,493
África	243,235	7,018	99,740
Sudáfrica	76,334	1,625	42,063
Oceanía	2,269	124	8,376
Australia	737	102	6,868

Note: Created by FUDECEN with information from Johns Hopkins University (2020).

COVID-19 will trigger a deep recession in the global economy. Oxford Economics (2020) estimates that the economy will slow down during the first semester of 2020 by -7% and then improve in the second semester. However, the severity of the crisis will cause permanent losses to the global economy. It is anticipated that the global GDP for 2020 will decrease by -2.8%. U.S. GDP will decline by -8%, China's by -12%, and the Eurozone will contract in the first quarter of 2020. The slowdown will lead to a reduction of trade, direct foreign investment, flows of tourism, remittances and key agricultural exports in the Central American region.

Figure 1 presents global economic estimates of the IMF (2020, a) which sustain that COVID-19 is inflicting high human costs worldwide and will seriously impact global economic activity (-3% in 2020), in a much worse scenario than the financial crisis of 2008–09.

The global economy, however, will be V-shaped and grow 5.8% in 2021.

Figure 1. Economic growth forecasts by region and for the U.S.

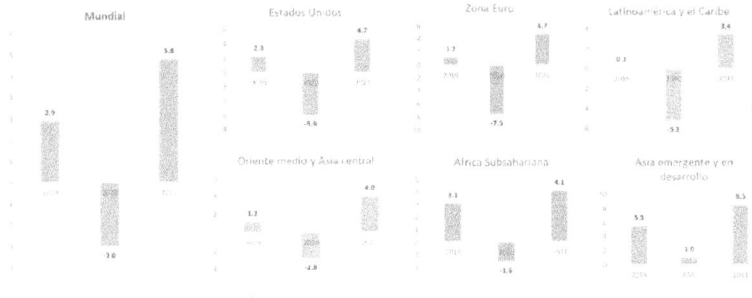

Note: Prepared by FUNDECEN with IMF data.

Of the various regions, emerging and developing Asia will best mitigate the pandemic's effects as it keeps its growth low though positive, near 1%, and in 2021 will expand to rates above 8%. This region will achieve the highest rates of growth.

The Eurozone is following the global trend, its growth plummeting -7.5% in 2020, but growing by 4.7% in 2021. Latin America follows as the second region with the greatest anticipated impact on its economic growth, its GDP growth rate declining by around 5%, while in 2021 a slight recovery of 3.4% is expected.

The Middle East and Central Asia together make up the third most strongly-hit region, with a growth deceleration of 2.8%, that will be recovered in 2021 until reaching a GDP growth rate of 4%. Sub-Saharan Africa is contracting slightly by -1.6% in 2020, and for 2021 will grow 4.1%. The U.S., El Salvador's primary trading partner, is expected to have a decline of -5.9% in 2020 and grow 4.7% in 2021.

In Central America, the countries experiencing the greatest deceleration in 2020 due to COVID-19 are: Nicaragua, -6.0%; El Salvador, -5.4%; Costa Rica, -3.3%; Honduras, -2.4%; Panama, -2.1%; Guatemala, -2.0%; and the Dominican Republic, -1.0%, the lowest in the region. It is anticipated that the highest rates of economic growth in 2021 will be registered by Guatemala (5.1%), Honduras (4.1%), the Dominican Republic and Panama (4.0%) (International Monetary Fund, 2020, a).

Main transmission channels of the impact of global deceleration in the El Salvadorian economy

In El Salvador's dollarized economy, monetary, credit and exchange policies have been removed since 2001 and fiscal policy action was limited until a credible fiscal policy was adopted. The result was the passing of a Fiscal Accountability Act in 2018. The dollarized monetary regime is more prone to crises in periods of global depression, such as the crisis occasioned by the COVID-19 pandemic. Since the dollarization, the crises of 2009 and 2020 have been successfully weathered, in part through a stage of fiscal self-determination followed by a period of fiscal consolidation, during which extreme fiscal austerity policies were put in place that resulted in the drastic reduction of disposable household income, high underemployment rates and migration to the U.S., where a third of the population now live. The global trade inventories of bulk goods, construction materials and commodities are contracting. Since the start of the crisis in China, the supply chain of intermediate goods has been disrupted and this will exert impacts on the Salvadoran economy. Cumulative imports of intermediate goods have declined as of April by -14.6% and the manufacturing industry by -15.7%, which explains the rate of decrease of the former.

The export demand from our principal partners, especially the U.S. (42% of exports) and Central America (47% of the export quota) is expected to fall.

In 2018 and 2019, exports of goods and services grew by 6.2% and 4.1%, respectively. The Central American Development Foundation (FUDECEN, 2020, b) foresees that in 2020 there will be a drop of -18% in exports of goods and services of and a decrease in CIF imports of -24%, despite the price reductions of crude oil and derivatives, in turn the consequence of approximately 30% less demand.

With regard to the channel of unilateral transfers of funds, the contribution of foreign remittances from relatives abroad to the Salvadoran economy amounts to US$ 4.4 billion, or 19% of the GDP between 2010 and 2018. A reduction of close to 17% is anticipated (International Monetary Fund, 2020) due to the slowing of economic activity in the U.S. and high unemployment in the month of May (18.9%) in the Hispanic population. The 2.5 million Salvadorans living abroad are in the precarious position of migrants without medical insurance, faced by the shutdowns of companies that employ them. Income from family remittances is expected to decline, which will affect approximately 20% of Salvadoran households.

With respect to finance and credit, El Salvador's risk rating is being upgraded to finance investments in the economy. The country's Standard and Poor's and Fitch risk ratings, are B-with a stable and negative outlook, a non-investment grade public debt rating. The Emerging Market Bond Index (EMBI) measures the difference between interest rates paid to dollar-denominated bonds, issued by underdeveloped countries, and U.S. Treasury Bonds, which are considered "risk-free". Two factors explain the evolution of country risk for El Salvador:

First, it is one of the emerging markets. Given the conditions of volatility in the financial markets caused by the pandemic, the Latin American EMBI had an increase in volatility from March 4 with a return of 3.72%, reaching a peak of 7.75% on March 23 with the exodus of investors from emerging markets, while the region's country risk has been gradually falling to 5.13% as of June 4.

Second, the country's internal conditions—the evolution of its economic growth, fiscal deficit and debt, joined with political stability. On March 4, the country risk reached a spread of 4.74% and continued to expand to its maximum of 9.91% on March 23. However, the country risk continued to increase until it reached 10.49% on May 20, which is explained by the failure of President Nayib Bukele to achieve a minimal consensus with the judiciary, the executive, and the social and productive sectors. There have been major violations of the Rule of Law that, according to Constitution, governs the country. One of them was the February 9 *coup d'état* that usurped the powers of the Legislative Branch and continues in power until the present. The country risk of sovereign bond issues in El Salvador reached a spread of 8.62 as of June 4, with 40% volatility, explained by internal factors.

Impacts expected on the population's living conditions and on aggregate supply and demand

The pandemic's effects on Salvadoran society are manifested in the increasing number of deaths and an exponential increase of COVID-19 infections, mainly in people with preexisting diabetes and hypertension, among other conditions, and an increased vulnerability of women and children. (See Figure 2).

Figure 2. Social impacts expected on the population

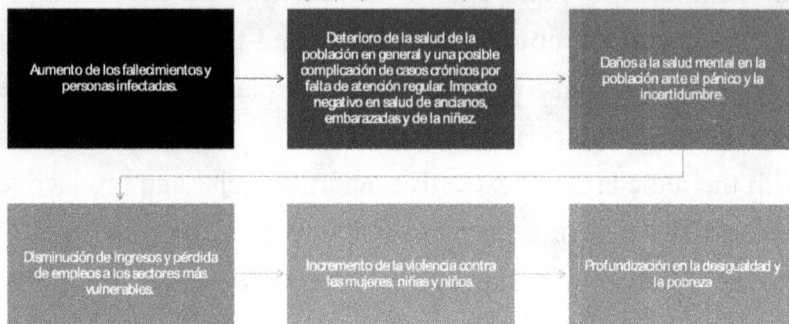

Note: Prepared by FUDECEN.

The government of El Salvador issued Executive Decree No. 4, declaring a "30-day quarantine after the declaration of the pandemic". Isolation was complete with the closure of airports, land and maritime customs facilities, to slow down the emergence of positive COVID-19 infections. Cases were detected eight days later in spite of the measures put in place; presumably the virus was already in the country. Several executive agreements extended the quarantine, which has now been in force longer than the quarantine of Wuhan, China.

The Legislative Assembly issued various decrees validating the state of national emergency and the state of public calamity and natural disaster caused by the COVID-19 virus (Asamblea Legislativa, 2020, a & b).

Figure 3. COVID-19 Case Figures

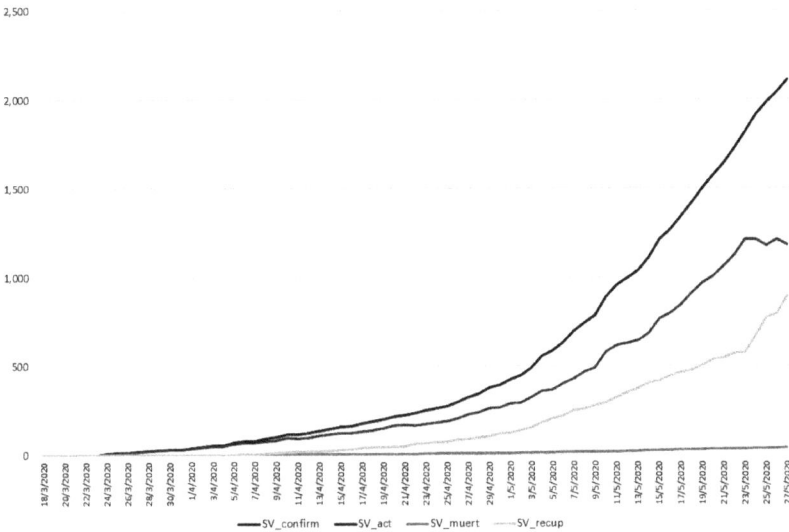

Note: Prepared by the authors with data from FUDECEN & NMD LATINOA-MÉRICA (2020).

Figure 3 shows the evolution of the pandemic in El Salvador. FUDECEN and NMD LATINOAMÉRICA (2020) have been publishing daily statistics on the number of confirmed, active, recovered cases and fatalities, and developing epidemiological models to facilitate public policy decision-making and save as many lives as possible. The numbers do not suggest that the COVID-19 outbreak is entering a stage of remission, as the reproductive number is greater than one (i.e., 1.6), meaning that each infected person is infecting at least one other person, despite the fact that the population has observed the quarantine, as documented by Google's Mobility Reports (2020). However, the reproductive number has remained stable at around 2 as the median, except for March 18 and 25, when it rose to a maximum of 9.

The Medical Association of El Salvador (2020) recommended the quarantine be maintained for 14 days, during which time the protocols of epidemiological surveillance had to be followed, and the approved biosafety protocols strictly complied with. FUNDAUNGO (2020, 10) developed an analytical tool of active cases, broken down according to the 262 municipalities in El Salvador. According to official statistics, 88 municipalities have recorded cases of COVID-19, while the other 174, on 66% of the national territory and where approximately 30% of the population live, have no active cases.

The policy of total lockdown implemented by the government did not segregate the vulnerable groups in the quarantine centers. For example, people over the age of 65, who make up 10% of the 2020 population, and among whom there is a greater prevalence of chronic diseases. As of 2019, 9% of this age group had diabetes (BID, 2020). Neither was there a separation of younger individuals with a propensity for developing cardiovascular disease, cancer, diabetes or COPD. A 2016 study found that 14% of 30 year olds were likely to die from these diseases before reaching the age of 70.

Figure 4. Basic reproductive number (R) as of May 31

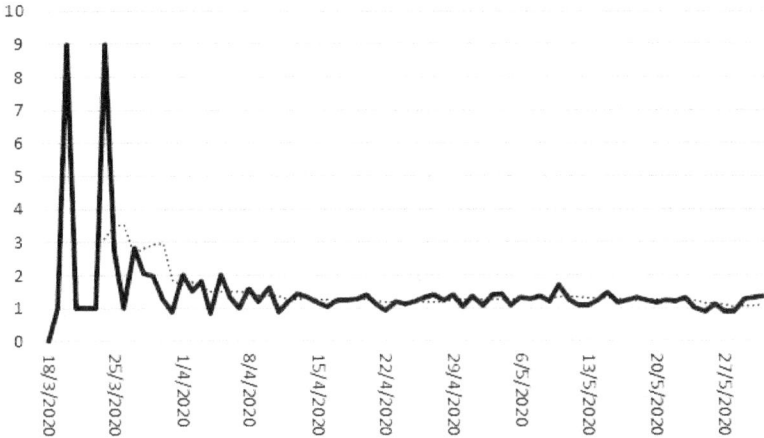

Note: Prepared by the authors with information from FUDECEN and NMD LATINOAMÉRICA (2020).

The intense political polarization created by the Executive has led to El Salvador's Constitutional Chamber of the Supreme Court of Justice (2020) to declare as unconstitutional Executive Decree Nos. 5, 12, 14, 18, 19, 21, 22, 24, 25, 26 and 29, Ministerial Resolution No. 101, and the Legislative Decree Nos. 611 and 639. The rationale put forth by the Constitutional Chamber for this ruling is that the Executive does not have the authority to impose limits on such fundamental rights as freedom of movement. However this power has been incorporated in the unilateral decrees for extending the duration of the mandatory quarantine and the Executive ordered the other two branches to work together on a bill to this effect. In summary, the El Salvador population has been under a mandatory quarantine for 85 days that was imposed through decrees that are not in strict adherence with the Constitution, and thus the country is now on the black list of nations that have responded to the crisis with excessive authoritarianism and overreach of the functions of other organs of the State. The mandatory quarantine has not flattened the curve; on the contrary, El Salvador is in a phase of expansion of the number of COVID-19 cases. In these conditions, on June 13 the government began to scale back the quarantine in five phases, with the final phase set to start on August 21. This series of measures leaves out 70% of workers, who are employed in the informal economy.

This external shock has created a current account deficit of approximately -5% of the GDP, and a decrease in the income from remittances. The government of El Salvador decided on a policy of increased spending in the face of falling tax revenues. To finance an estimated fiscal deficit of -13.9% of the GDP, financing in the amount of US$3,000 was obtained through credits from international organizations and bond issues.

The Impacts

In terms of the expected social impacts on Salvadoran families, in income terms poverty will rise from 28% to 39% and 600,000 more persons will live below the poverty line. This means that the middle class will shrink from 22% to 17%. (BID, 2020, p. 20). The estimates of impact on employment in 2020, according to FUDECEN (2020, b) range from a loss of 240,800 jobs in a scenario of short-term crisis, to a prolonged recession that would cost 669,200 jobs. The hardest hit sectors will be businesses, restaurants and hotels, the service sector and the manufacturing industry. Growth will fall-7.2% in 2020 and rise 3.1% in 2021.

Given the financial instability in the dollarized economy caused by the external shock during 2020, public policy makers will be subsequently inclined to establish plans for fiscal consolidation, given that the ratios exceed the limits set by the Fiscal Accountability Act for Public Financial Sustainability.

Central America: A Look at Public Policy for the Attenuation of the Infection Curve

Fitch Ratings and the IMF (2020, b, p. 3) analyzed the evolution of health care systems in the Latin American region, mentioning that in Central America, Panama, the Dominican Republic, Costa Rica and El Salvador are better prepared in terms of health indicators to face the pandemic than Honduras, Nicaragua and Guatemala (See Figure 5).

The countries of the Central American Integration System (*Sistema para la Integración Centroamericana*, SICA) initiated their confinement measures in the first half of March. El Salvador and Honduras imposed a total quarantine, while Belize, Costa Rica, Guatemala, the Dominican Republic and Panama implemented partial social distancing measures. Nicaragua did not impose any measures.

On March 12, the presidents of Honduras, Costa Rica, Guatemala, Nicaragua, Panama, the Dominican Republic and the deputy prime minister of Belize adopted a Regional Contingency Plan incorporating five pillars: 1) Health and Risk Management, 2) Business and Finance, 3) Security, Justice and Migration, 4) Strategic Communications, and 5) Management of International Cooperation. The plan adds transversal considerations, such as food and nutritional security, the role of micro-, small-and medium-sized enterprises (*Micro, Pequeñas y Medianas Empresas*, MIPYME), and the gender perspective for the protection of women's rights (*Sistema de Integración Centroaméricana*, SICA, 2020).

Figure 5. Latin America: Selected Health Care Statistics

Latin America Pandemic Vulnerability Matrix
Key Strengths & Vulnerabilities By Category

	Global Health Security Index Score	Doctors (Per 100,000 Population)	Hospital Beds (Per 100,000 Population)	Total Government Debt, % of GDP, 2020f	Budget Balance, % of GDP, 2020f
Argentina	58.6	39.6	50	89.5	-4.5
Bolivia	35.8	16.11	11	50.0	-7.3
Brazil	59.7	21.5	22	81.8	-6.0
Chile	58.3	10.8	22	29.5	-4.0
Colombia	44.2	20.84	15	46.1	-2.3
Costa Rica	45.1	11.5	11.6	63.4	-5.7
Ecuador	50.1	20.5	15	40.7	-2.6
El Salvador	44.2	15.69	13	74.3	-3.2
Guatemala	32.7	3.55	6	25.2	-2.3
Guayana	31.7	7.99	16	54.6	-2.5
Honduras	27.6	3.14	7	42.2	-2.7
Mexico	57.6	22.48	15.2	49.9	-2.3
Nicaragua	43.1	10.06	9	58.4	-3.6
Panama	43.7	15.7	23	39.9	-2.5
Paraguay	35.7	13.66	13	25.0	-3.0
Peru	49.2	12.7	16	25.0	-1.9
Suriname	36.5	12.27	31	56.1	-4.5
Uruguay	41.3	50.5	28	66.4	-3.6
Venezuela	23	19.24	8	N/A	-25.3

Note: This matrix is not a ranking of the countries as the categories are not scored or weighted. Source: NTI, JHU, WHO, Fitch Solutions

Note: Prepared by the authors with information from FITCH Ratings, 2020).

The plan enables the SICA countries to access funds amounting to over US$1.9 billion, $1 billion for the Central Bank Support Contingency Fund (*Fondo Contingente de apoyo a Bancos Centrales*), US$550 million for the Fiscal Emergency Fund (*Fondo de Emergencia Fiscal*) and US$350 million for a liquidity program for the commercial banking sector of the SICA countries.

Figure 6. Central America: Number of COVID-19 cases

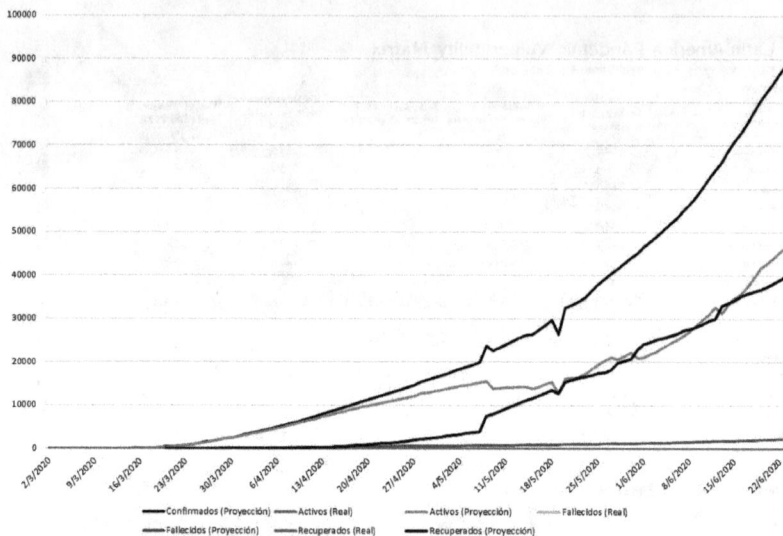

Note: Prepared by the authors with information from FUDECEN & NMD LATINOAMÉRICA (2020).

Figure 6 shows the evolution of COVID-19 cases in the member countries of the Central American Integration System (SICA), where as of June 20, 2020 the number of active cases reached 40,389, the number of recovered cases 35,972, and the number of deaths, 2,064 (FUDECEN & NMD LATINOAMÉRICA, 2020).

The cases in the Central American region are still in a phase of accelerated propagation in Guatemala, Costa Rica and Honduras, while in El Salvador, Panama, the Dominican Republic and Belize, the number of recovered cases exceeds that of active cases, to form an "X" graph as of June 20 (FUDECEN & NMD LATINOAMÉRICA, 2020)(FUDECEN, 2020, c).

Once the COVID-19 infection curve flattens, a dialog must be established with the different social actors in the Central American Region in order to transition from a development model that has created large gaps of territorial inequality, lack of human opportunities, and social exclusion, toward a new model of a knowledge-based, diversified and modern society that can transform the productive structure into complex goods and services, generate decent employment and enable its citizens to enjoy good quality of life. The prescribed economic policy is to reach agreement on an Inclusive Pro-Growth Agenda, based on the expansion of effective demand and structural transformation. This will be achieved by implementing policies that are stable over time, but also flexible enough to adapt to changing economic conditions. Policies should be endowed with enough stability and credibility, and to this end it is important to avoid resorting to excessively inflexible and inefficient regulations. We propose the following: "Inter-temporal agreements are the mechanism that can prevent the abuse of political power by an incumbent. In such a context the political power game will be more cooperative in character and lead to public policy formulation that can be more effective, sustainable and flexible in response to changes in economic or social conditions" (Scartascini et al., 2010, p. 6).

China and support for Central America during the pandemic

Amid this scenario, China's presence has clearly acquired new significance, if one compares her diplomatic ties with the region and the Caribbean in the past, to those of the present. China's recent proposals have emphasized the vision of "a global community with a shared future", with all the countries working together, sharing objective scientific research on COVID-19 viral infection, pathogenesis, transmission routes and transmissibility, in order to contain the spread of the virus and protect the health and well-being of people around the world. Assistance to the Central American region and the Caribbean has been promoted with the countries that maintain diplomatic relations with China.

On June 5, 2020, President Xi JinPing had a telephone conversation with the president of Costa Rica, Carlos Alvarado. It was one of several phone calls and/or meetings between around 50 foreign leaders and heads of international organizations and the Chinese president, to share China's tactical actions and achievements in the fight against the virus, and to emphasize China's open, transparent and responsible approach to the dissemination of information and sharing her experience of controlling and treating infected cases.

The conversation with the president of Costa Rica concerned the impact of the COVID-19 pandemic and the support offered in these circumstances, especially in the form of medical supplies. President Xi mentioned in this respect that China would continue to firmly safeguard equality and international justice and the legitimate rights and interests of small and mid-sized developing countries. China is prepared to work with Costa Rica to strengthen international cooperation for the united resistance against the epidemic, safeguard the developing countries' anti-epidemic efforts and global public health security.

President Carlos Alvarado said that, since the establishment of diplomatic ties 13 years ago between Costa Rica and China, the friendship between the two countries has progressively deepened and their mutually beneficial cooperation has continued to expand. In an official communique the Costa Rica government expressed its firm adherence to the principle of One China, and that it is willing to strengthen exchanges and cooperation with China in public health, infrastructure, culture and other fields, to become a bridge and a port of entry into Central America, to move the relations between Costa Rica and China forward to a new stage. During their conversation, the Costa Rican president welcomed President Xi Jinping's announcement that the vaccine developed by China will be employed as an international public good immediately it becomes available.

The Chinese government sent 50 tons of equipment to Costa Rica, including 726,000 units of personal protection equipment for health workers. Panama as well has benefited from the joint efforts of the Chinese public and private sectors, and of Panama's Chinese community, to mobilize basic food supplies and the technology for the speedy diagnosis of patients with COVID-19. In El Salvador, in the early stages of the outbreak, China donated a consignment of 100,000 masks, 10,080 test kits and five ventilators.

The Dominican Republic received an initial donation of supplies from the Chinese government valued at US$ 100,000 to assist local efforts to combat the coronavirus pandemic. The materials included disposable protective medical clothing, medical goggles, infrared hand thermometers for measuring forehead temperature, protective face masks for medical use, pairs of sterile disposable rubber surgical gloves, and insulating medical shoe covers.

The Chinese private sector and the local Chinese community in the Dominican Republic have deployed assistance throughout the country. COVID-19 test kits from the Hefei Institute for Public Safety Research at Tsinghua University, masks and test kits, as well as four ventilators have been provided.

The Dominican Republic, Costa Rica, Panama and El Salvador have received scientific cooperation assistance from the Chinese government and experts in the management of COVID-19 cases, to share experiences in researching virus traceability, medicines, vaccines and tests, scientific research data and information. They have done a joint study of strategies of prevention, control and treatment. The foregoing is of course also framed in the context of the new diplomatic relations that China has successfully consolidated in Central America and the Caribbean, upon transforming a situation that was adverse for her in the past. It goes without saying that the Central American countries are aware that their future will be marked by tensions that may arise from differences between Washington and Beijing; however, they hope to successfully navigate those rough waters with a modicum of balance.

VII. Cuba's Experience: Combating the COVID-19 Pandemic

Ambassador Pedro Monzón Barata[1]

We are still in the middle of the pandemic and so it's difficult to predict the future. But everything seems to indicate that the changes taking place in Cuba will serve to better detect the health markers of the disease and ascertain the status of its spread in the country.

Cuba's successes in fighting the pandemic have been essentially conditioned on the radical changes that were ushered in and took root with the triumph of the 1959 Revolution.

Contrary to what occurred in many countries with the imposition of neoliberalism, the Cuban State grew strong and became the owner of most of the nation's means of production and resources. This ensured the putting into practice of strategies that prioritized development and social policies based on socialist concepts, in which humanism plays an essential role. With this degree of state support and based on these policies, substantial funding has been channeled to fundamental economic sectors, public health, education, the sciences and culture.

1. Researcher at the Center for International Policy Research (Centro de Investigaciones de Política Internacional, CIPI).

These national policies rest on two essential pillars: independence and social justice, which also underpin foreign policy and explain Cuba's behavior in response to the novel coronavirus pandemic.

Domestic and foreign policy rest on the principles of sovereignty and self-determination. No foreign country or organization can impose outside concepts that ignore these precepts, which are at the heart of development and national security. Nevertheless, Cuba has indeed assimilated everything that can strengthen the country's interests and is aligned with the established international norms. Thus, Cuba observes the international laws and mandates of such institutions as the WHO, even as she rejects the imposition of models such as those that come from the IMF, that engender destitution and other serious social hardships.

In a 2020 paper published by the Cuban Academic Journal of Sciences (*Revista de la Academia de Ciencias de Cuba*), Cuban President Miguel Díaz-Canel Bermúdez asserted that over 27% of the national budget is allocated to health care and social welfare costs. The national budget guarantees essential public services and sufficient food for the population, in spite of difficulties emanating from the U.S. trade embargo. The focus on feeding the people is so effective that the FAO has recognized that hunger has been eradicated on the island and UNICEF does not detect any childhood malnutrition, a key indicator of citizen welfare (*Oficina Regional de la FAO para América Latina y el Caribe; Fondo de las Naciones Unidas para la Infancia*, UNICEF).

Because health care and education are the property of the citizens, they have provided the people of Cuba with free, universal, standardized and high quality services for over half a century. This has ensured a high level of science and education and a healthy population, with indicators that rank above global averages, such that Cuba stacks up favorably even alongside the developed countries.

The health care and the education systems provide coverage from one extreme of the country to the other, including the most remote areas, and are designed to serve the entire population, not merely the affluent social groups. Thus, according to Infomed, the web portal of the Cuban Ministry of Public Health, Cuba has the largest number of doctors per capita in the world (nine for every 1,000 persons), beds per capita (5.8) are double the global average, and hospitals, outpatient clinics and general practitioners abound, all strengths that stand alongside other logistical and human advantages. The education of health care workers-doctors, nurses, technicians-is based on values and on primary care, preventive, and community-based medicine, without detriment to excellence in training for the cure of disease. To train all of these health care human resources, Cuba has 13 universities and nine medical science schools, four dental schools, one nursing school, one health technology school, three technology and nursing schools, 12 medical science campuses, the Latin American School of Medicine, and the National School of Public Health (Díaz-Canel, op. cit.).

Robust Science Hubs

A mainstay of public health policy has been the creation of cutting-edge science hubs for biotechnology and pharmacy. We have available drugs that are of high scientific value and have great efficacy for treating many diseases, which have armed the fight against COVID-19 in Cuba and in countries that benefit from our collaboration. Thanks to the system that is in place, the Cuban State has invested large funds in advances in these sectors, whose development require long periods of time. Such an endeavor would have been very difficult to accomplish had it relied on private interests, which prioritize quick returns from earnings.

The Cuban science hub also generates exportable goods and services and advanced technologies in food production, ensuring high quality standards, according to reports from the Genetic Engineering and Biotechnology Center (*Centro de Ingeniería Genética y Biotecnología*, CIGB). It is essential to highlight that with respect to clinical trials for any new product or, for example, a novel vaccine, these research agencies coordinate seamlessly with all institutions directly or indirectly linked to health care in Cuba, and that are state run. This speeds up the achievement of results and significantly cuts down on costs.

At present, the Cuban science hub consists of 32 companies with 65 basic business units (*unidades empresariales de base*), 80 production lines, and 21 associated science and technology units. Its human capital consists of over 20,000 workers with an average age of 42 years. Seventeen thousand of them are professionals, technicians and operators. This workforce includes 1,265 people with master's degrees and 278 Doctors of Science. The system generates hundreds of medications and products, many of them unique to Cuba, such as the lung cancer vaccine, specific treatments for other types of cancer, Heberprot-P, which prevents amputation of the lower extremities in diabetic patients, diverse drugs that boost the human immune system, retrovirals and others for the treatment of vitiligo, psoriasis, etc. (Biocubafarma, op. cit.).

Thus, the conditions created in Cuba to tackle the pandemic are not the result of improvisation in front of an extremely serious public health emergency, such as the current one we are facing. On the other hand, a health system with such attributes (that benefits other branches of science and the economy as well) has been a guarantee of the nation's sovereignty in this important sector. This acquires special significance in light of the conditions of economic, trade, and financial embargo that Cuba has been subjected to for decades.

It should be added that, alongside the achievement of generally high and consistent levels of education that began with the literacy education of the entire population in 1961, Cuba implemented a cultural policy throughout the national territory. For this reason, the majority of the population is able to understand, make a commitment to, and participate as a protagonist of national policies, especially those referred to health issues. Throughout the pandemic, although there have indeed been episodes of undesirable lack of discipline, albeit minor ones, and many due to supply problems caused by the embargo, the people have been kept closely informed of the pandemic's spread in the country, what measures had to be taken, and they have generally followed the national guidelines.

This entire complex of factors becomes integrated, when the circumstances so require, in a single institutional system that gathers together grassroots and political organizations with large memberships, extensive reach and popular influence, representing the interests of a broad swath of the population and channeling their social participation; media outlets that are state-owned and adhere to guidelines that are essentially educational, cultural, and political; governmental bodies at the provincial and municipal levels; universities, research centers, trade organizations, etc. They are all interconnected in a proactive manner with the policy-making centers, with which they interact, above all in exceptional circumstances, such as a natural disaster or an epidemic. This system has been tested time and again as part of the Civil Defense, which explains the country's positive outcomes in dealing with the hurricanes that are quite common in this part of the world, and with epidemics.

It must be stated that for this system to work properly, it has been fundamental for there to be ongoing direct dialog between scientists, experts, academics and professionals and the government; the fostering of inter-agency and inter-sectoral cooperation; interdisciplinary work; the deployment of intense efforts to accelerate response times, and active public outreach for improved information and response on the part of the population (Díaz-Canel, op.cit.).

Actions and Decisions

Thanks to this system, during the pandemic a cascade of decisions and actions were rolled out, of which we cite just a few:
• Daily broadcasts of orientation and information to the general public via television and the press, in great detail and including causal assessments of the disease in the country, including how many people were tested, how many were symptomatic, pre-

symptomatic and asymptomatic; numbers of hospitalized, those who had recovered, patients in critical and serious condition, and deaths.

• Measures adopted at the national, provincial, municipal and neighborhood level of social isolation or quarantining, depending on the evolution of the local situation.

• Design and execution of mass testing, door-to-door, carried out by approximately 30,000 medical students and, in lesser numbers, by social workers. This enabled detecting the people who were sick, pre-symptomatic and asymptomatic-essential information for the containment of infection.

• Public transportation use was restricted to 50% of normal capacity and mask-wearing was made mandatory.

• No one has been cut off salary wise; efforts have been made to ensure access to a basic basket of food and hygiene products, despite the enormous constraints imposed by the embargo and the added economic hardship created by the pandemic.

• As is customary, the entire Cuban population has been assured of free medical and dental care. The prison system has its own hospitals, social welfare centers and outposts, and its own doctors.

• The activities vital for the country to keep functioning were continued, following strict protective guidelines, other activities were supported by working remotely, classes were continued via television and virtual sales shot up

(Díaz-Canel, op.cit.; Daily nationwide TV newscasts on the pandemic Dr. Alberto Durán García).

Many other actions of a technical and scientific nature were carried out, as follows:

• Mathematical models were developed and updated to enable predicting, resolving and evaluating the pandemic's evolution, and a geolocation system was used to assist in epidemiological management;

• Biomarkers were studied to forecast the severity of the disease; zones of clinical and epidemiological risk were mapped, locating at-risk groups of persons aged 60 years and older throughout the country;

• The Cuban-designed ultra-micro-analytical system (*Sistema ultra-micro-analítico cubano*, SUMA) was used as a diagnostic method for testing the population;

• Protective equipment was developed and manufactured for health care workers; Cuban prototypes of emergency ventilators were designed and developed;

• An ultra-violet disinfection light was designed and developed;

• Big data techniques were used to make assessments of the population's mobility during the proliferation of the disease;

• The Public Health Ministry began a research study on seroprevalence (the presence of antibodies) and the prevalence of COVID-19 in Cuba, in accordance with WHO recommendations.

• Clinical trials were conducted for the treatment of critical and acutely-ill patients;

• The Cuban Clinical-Epidemiological Management Model to Combat and Control COVID-19 (*Modelo cubano de gestión Clínico-epidemiológica para el Enfrentamiento y Control de la COVID-19*) was developed and implemented.

• As of mid-June, 460 research studies as part of the COVID-19 research plan had been carried out. On average, each week there are 8.3 studies and medical products, equipment, and devices that are analyzed and approved for development in Cuba.

• The social sciences have participated in impact mitigation, collective co-responsibility for care, the participation of individuals and of communities, and innovative initiatives for dealing with isolation.

• Multi-level and artificial intelligence models were developed to make comparisons of the epidemic's behavior in Cuba and in other countries in the region and throughout the world; to predict the epidemic's end and post-epidemic behavior, and to design programs for mental health intervention and psychological support to cope with the COVID-19 pandemic (Díaz-Canel, op.cit.).

• The National Genetics Group (*Grupo Nacional de Genética*) conducted a study on genetic predisposition to COVID-19, in alignment with other international research studies demonstrating that blood-type A persons were more likely to acquire COVID-19, and showing a propensity in persons with

Blood Type A to contract the virus and develop complications. Progress has been made on this study, initial results have been achieved, making it possible to tailor treatments to the genetic characteristics of each patient.

• Thirty major drugs to treat COVID-19 have been produced, including antivirals, antiarrhythmics, antibiotics, and immunizing agents to treat complications in the sick who get infected with COVID-19.

• Recombinant Alpha 2b Interferon and its combination with Gamma Interferon have been used successfully in Cuba, China, and other countries.

• Cuba has also begun using other medications that boost the immune system. Five major Cuban vaccine candidates have also been developed, in addition to the monoclonal antibody Anti-CD6, the peptide CIGB258 (Jusvinza), and HeberFeron for COVID-19 patients, Biomodulin-T, and a homeopathic drug (Preven-gHo Vir) for senior citizens living in long-term care facilities.

• The Cuban vaccine for meningitis, Va Mengoc BC, has been administered to boost the immune system capacity of patients and medical staff.

• National conditions were created for the production of the anti-retroviral Kaletra (which has been a worldwide success), currently used in the Cuban treatment protocol.

• All of these tools were applied to the creation of a national treatment protocol, adapted to the requirements as the concrete circumstances have evolved (Díaz-Canel op.cit.; Daily nationwide TV newscasts on the pandemic by Dr. Alberto Durán García).

A brief description follows of some important Cuban products used to treat the disease.

PRODUCTOS DE LA INDUSTRIA BIOFARMACÉUTICA CUBANA PARA EL TRATAMIENTO DE LA COVID-19

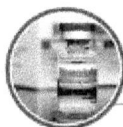

BIOMODULINA T

Este medicamento ya se ha aplicado en más de 8 000 ancianos, quienes dieron su consentimiento informado, y solo se reportan 14 reacciones adversas. Hay una reducción en más del 40% de los eventos de infecciones respiratorias agudas, así como disminuyó los ingresos hospitalarios y la mortalidad asociada a este padecimiento.

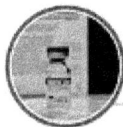

INTERFERÓN ALFA 2 B HUMANO RECOMBINANTE

Tiene la capacidad de interferir la multiplicación viral dentro de la célula. Este fármaco es capaz de cubrir la deficiencia de producción natural de interferón que provoca el SARS-CoV-2, fortaleciendo el sistema inmunológico. Al cuarto día de ser utilizado el interferón en los pacientes con la COVID-19 en Cuba, un 37 % de los casos había eliminado el virus y a los siete días, el 78 %.

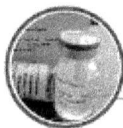

ITOLIZUMAB

El ensayo clínico del anticuerpo monoclonal ha abarcado a 10 hospitales de La Habana y de varias provincias, con una muestra de más de 70 pacientes, con una edad promedio de 69 años, el primero fue tratado el 28 de marzo. La tasa global de mejoría del distrés respiratorio fue del 70 %; en el caso de los pacientes graves fue del 90 %, con una tasa de supervivencia del 80 %, que llegó a ser del 87.5 % en el caso de los pacientes con enfermedad moderada.

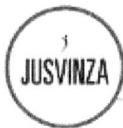

JUSVINZA (CIGB 258)

Tiene características inmunoreguladoras y ha sido utilizado con éxito en la atención a pacientes con artritis reumatoidea. La supervivencia en los pacientes críticos con COVID-19 fue del 73.7 % y en los graves del 91. 3 %, con un promedio de casi 86 %. Los resultados apuntan a que el péptido es capaz de modular la inflamación y no ocurre una inmunosupresión marcada, no hay focos de fibrosis, lo cual contribuye a la calidad de vida posterior de los pacientes.

CUBADEBATE

These products explain Cuba's positive outcomes in fighting the pandemic. Cuba is one of the countries with the best indicators in the world, the least number of people infected, the highest percentage of recovery (nearly 95%), a critical reduction in deaths, and prevention of health care system collapse.

In other words, as this paper was concluded, in Cuba the number of infected persons had fallen substantially, hospital admissions had gone down to a minimum, and the death toll had stopped rising. The overall care program and Cuban biotechnology products explain this phenomenon, above all the critical reduction of deaths. While Cuba is saving 80% of critical and acutely ill patients, a figure that is rising by the day; in the rest of the world 80% of patients are being lost. At this time, Cuba's mortality rate is lower than that of the rest of the world and of the Americas. This figure should continue to decline given that the number of deaths is decreasing. Thus, as of June 15, Cuba's mortality rate was 0.74, while for the 20 countries selected from the Americas and included in this work, the mean is 6.57 (Díaz-Canel op.cit., Statista; COVID-19 mortality rate in selected Latin American and Caribbean countries as of June 15, 2020, per 100,000 inhabitants; Dr. Alberto Durán Garcia, daily TV newscasts).

Despite continuing exposure to the disease, thanks to the mechanisms of protection and immunization administered to the staff there have been null mortalities among health care workers.

Neither have there been any deaths in the prisons, thanks to the specialized care given to the prisoners. During this time period, protection measures will remain in effect to prevent a new outbreak of the epidemic.

As shown in the following graph, the behavior of the disease is stable and this is expected to continue, the projection being that it will be trending favorably.

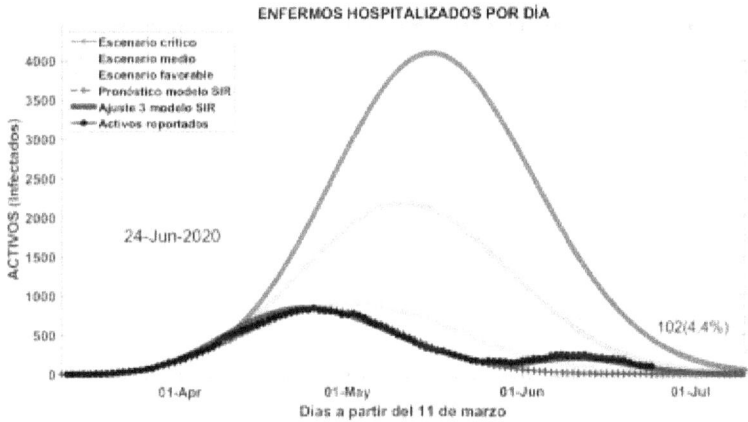

ENFERMOS HOSPITALIZADOS POR DÍA

Source: Dr. Alberto Durán García, Director of Epidemiology, Cuban Ministry of Public Health, in charge of reporting daily to the public on the pandemic.

Cuban Foreign Policy and Medical Solidarity

Within the sphere of foreign policy, Cuba's role in the pandemic has been oriented by solidarity. Her behavior in response to the pandemic has been consistent with this tradition.

The Henry Reeve Medical Brigade (*Contingente Henry Reeve*) has provided assistance in disaster events and severe epidemics since its beginnings, and has been deployed to over 30 countries. Over 2,000 highly trained and experienced medical doctors are members of its medical contingents. The medical brigades have extended their services in solidarity with nations whose governments have requested their help, including developed countries such as Italy, the Principality of Andorra and France.

These expert medical units have been joined by another 28,000 doctors who were already working in 61 countries. Although the Henry Reeve Brigade has received little media attention, since its founding it has accumulated a long trajectory of international cooperation in over 28 countries, including Guatemala, Pakistan, Bolivia, Ecuador, Indonesia, Peru, Mexico, China, Chile, Haiti, Sierra Leone, Guinea, Liberia (to fight Ebola), Nepal, Dominica, Venezuela, Nicaragua, Suriname, Jamaica, Haiti, Italy, Andorra, Spain, and Martinique, an overseas region and Department of France (Díaz-Canel, op. cit.; Cuba-debate, Granma).

The brigades' missions all deal with highly infectious, high-risk disease outbreaks, often in impoverished, hard-to-reach areas, in conditions of disaster where the inhabitants spoke other languages and whose cultures were very different from Cuban culture. On many occasions extreme effort was required.

The Brigade was founded in 2005 by the leader of the

Cuban Revolution, Fidel Castro, with an initial membership of 1,500 health care workers. It now has over 7,000 members. Membership is voluntary, based on a sense of vocation and personal conviction, and the volunteers go through ethics training. Aside from their backgrounds as doctors, members have knowledge of epidemiology and catastrophe-related diseases; they must speak two foreign languages, be in good physical condition and possess the necessary training and willingness to rapidly deploy to wherever they are needed. Like all Cuban doctors they are trained to prioritize primary and community health care and preventive medicine (Díaz-Canel, op. cit., Cubadebate, Periódico Granma).

For all the above reasons and after having received many international awards, in 2017 the Brigade was granted the Lee Jong-wook Memorial Prize for Public Health from the WHO. Also, at this time a major worldwide campaign is underway with the support of governments, associations, institutions, and renowned personalities for the Brigade's nomination to be awarded the Nobel Peace Prize. Neither Cuba nor the Cuban doctors render services for economic, ideological or political gain, to receive awards or any other type of public recognition; they do so purely for humanitarian reasons. Nevertheless, the reasons are many that explain the worthiness of honoring the brigade, on the part of various quarters in the world.

Aside from those already mentioned, the following can

be said by way of a summary: the work done by the Brigade, its special character worldwide, the tangible results in healing many thousands of people and the prevention of loss of life in many countries. Considering the needs of today's world population, there is a lack of millions of doctors, and many already practicing physicians work in an urban setting and have no interest in assuming sacrifices and risks. In contrast, the Cuban Brigade serves in underdeveloped areas, often in far-flung disaster-hit locations. The Cuban doctors who are Brigade members run great risks, as in the campaign against Ebola. Another important goal of all who support the nomination is that, upon publicly acknowledging the brigades' sacrifices, effectiveness, and the quality of their work, a stop can be put to the media manipulation, statements and actions of U.S. government officials against the Cuban medical assistance campaigns (Cubadebate; Ecured).

Below is a map of the Brigade's deployment in different countries of the world, which has to be updated almost weekly.

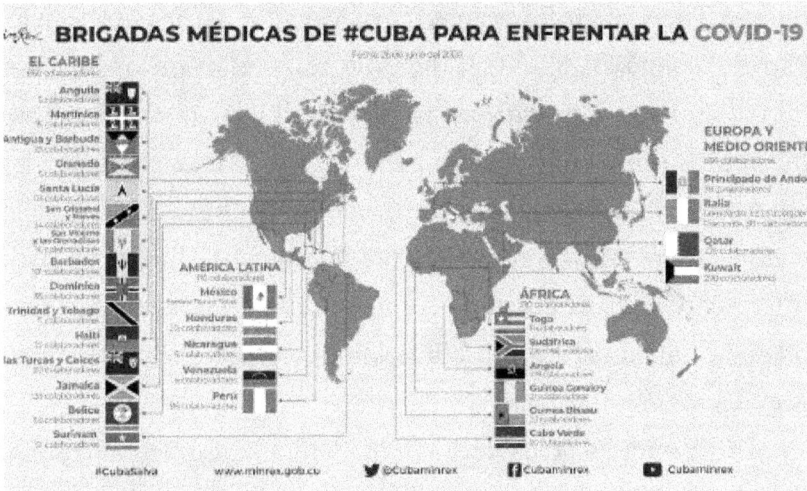

Source: CUBAMINREX CUBA, June 26, 2020.

China-Cuba Cooperation in the Fight against the Pandemic

As part of this national effort and international solidarity, Cuba has received the backing and been accompanied by the People's Republic of China in an exemplary reciprocity and partnership.

The Caribbean island closely followed the unfolding events and offered, from the first, its modest contribution to the Asian giant in light of the devastating effects of the pandemic. A Cuban medical brigade took part in this effort and a Cuban antiviral, Interferon Alpha-2b, was included in the suite of products with which China combated the symptoms of the illness. The Cuban Foreign Affairs Minister, Bruno Rodriguez Parrilla, acknowledged that the drug was the result of bilateral biotechnology innovation, as it is produced in Changchun, through a joint venture company of the two countries. The enterprise is associated with other joint companies on the continent and will soon include the first binational biotech park for researching, developing, producing and marketing Cuban pharmaceuticals of proven efficacy and world renown (Granma, May 13, 2020).

Dr. Yamira Palacios, Head of the Office of Comercializadora de Servicios Médicos S.A. and leader of the China Mission in charge of Cuban cooperation, announced: "We will continue contributing to societal welfare and quality of life together with our Chinese brothers and sisters who are doctors and health care workers and models of hard work, courage and dedication." The statement is indicative of the bonds of fellowship that already exist between the experts of the two countries (Granma, July 10, 2020).

Cuba has always shown admiration for how China has managed the pandemic and noted the importance of her experience for designing the Cuban campaign. The Cuban ambassador to Beijing, Carlos Miguel Pereira Hernández, declared, "Cuba has consistently recognized the validity of China's efforts in extremis to contain the virus.... Nothing was left to chance, although there are still voices who insist on spreading blame and imputations of criminal conduct on social media. Every single experience was studied and reflected on endlessly...."

China's example was followed and studied by the Cuban authorities and scientists who designed and implemented their own strategy early on: "With her comprehensive approach to the epidemic outbreak, informative transparency, and the decisive role played by her scientific institutions, China offered us a paradigm that we could adapt to our nation's reality and possibilities. And did so with the greatest integrity, without hesitation or exaggeration, in a cool and calm manner; and yet again defending the inalienable premise that in our country, health is a human right for all that has been won," the Cuban ambassador sustained (Granma, July 10, 2020).

The assistance given by China to Cuba did not stop at offering a model of how to fight the disease, but was also concretized in the form of essential donations. Aside from the exemplary assistance provided to many other countries around the world, China sent donations to Cuba in April and May of supplies to fight coronavirus. The donors included various ministries, government agencies and the Communist Party of China, the Foreign Affairs Office of Henan, as well as the companies SKN, Xiamen Carisol, Yutong, Geely, Beijing Rosa, BPL, Changheber, Shanghai Suncuba, and Beya Time, among others. The donations consisted of ordinary and surgical face masks, disposable protective suits, infrared thermometers, protective goggles, surgical gloves and shoe covers. At the official handover ceremony held at the headquarters of the Ministry of Public Health of Cuba, the Ambassador of the People's Republic of China to Cuba, Chen Xi, emphasized that the two nations are brothers and their solidarity will continue in spite of these difficult times.

The Chinese Embassy in Havana also donated US$ 200,000 dollars to the Cuban health authorities and gave assurances that further donations were planned. At the event, the Chinese ambassador recognized the Cuban State and People's fight against the pandemic and confirmed the mutual solidarity that has informed their two nations' bilateral relations for six decades. "This coronavirus knows nothing of borders or nationalities. Only through mutual support can we protect ourselves. This is why both Cuba and China share their rejection of the pandemic's politicization and stigmatization, which has already cost so many lives. Our nation has gradually defeated COVID-19 and we are sure that Cuba will, too, thanks to the actions of her government and the discipline of her people," he pointed out. For his part, the Deputy Chief of the Department of International Relations of the Central Committee of the Cuban Communist Party, Ángel Arzuaga Reyes, who also took part in the ceremony, expressed thanks for the gesture of solidarity. "At a time when the U.S. government is ramping up its cruel and genocidal economic, trade, and financial embargo against our country, and blocking our ability to purchase and transport the supplies we need to fight SARS-CoV-2, Cuba and China have become referents of cooperation based on equality and mutual respect" (Granma, April 24 & May 13, 2020).

Another donation was made by appreciative former Chinese students of Cuban educational institutions and by Chinese companies based in Havana. However, a donation by Jack Ma, the founder of the Chinese electronics giant Alibaba, consisting of masks, fast diagnostic kits and ventilators, was blocked by the U.S. embargo, and the plane transporting the consignment was prevented from landing in Havana.

In February, Cuban President Miguel Díaz-Canel recognized the gestures of Chinese solidarity in a conversation with President Xi Jinpin. During the dialog across the distance, President Xi observed that, after the disease broke out, Army General Raúl Castro Ruz, First Secretary of the Central Committee of the Cuban Communist Party, and President Díaz-Canel immediately expressed their solidarity to the Chinese head of state, and Cuba's president also made a special visit to the Chinese Embassy on the island to reaffirm his support (Granma, July 10, 2020).

Cuba was the first country in Latin America to establish diplomatic ties with China, in 1960. Since then, the relationship has been conducted at the highest official levels, and has now been manifested during the pandemic. The two countries uphold and agree on a policy of full support for multilateralism, in opposition to hegemonism, interventionism and all violations of the U.N. Charter and the principles of international law. For her part, China is firmly opposed to the economic, trade, and financial embargo imposed on Cuba by the U.S.

The Embargo and the Attack on Public Health

Against the backdrop of China's noble international humanitarian actions based on the policy of solidarity, far from emulating this example or simply respectfully acknowledging it, the U.S. instead launched an intense media offensive to discredit China with racist and xenophobic messages, and blamed the country for triggering the pandemic. Cuba, naturally, has supported China, debunking the falsehoods. The U.S. has sought to cover up its own national disaster that resulted from poor management of the disease, to prevent China from consolidating the position of international moral leadership that she has won during the awaited post-pandemic "new normal"; to seek the support of U.S. voters in the upcoming elections and pump up the Trump administration's motto of "America First." As part of the campaign aspiring to global dominance, the U.S. has attacked the WHO and multilateralism in general, the trend that the administration has fomented since its inauguration.

The purpose behind the aggressive U.S. policy of continuing the trade blockade against Cuba has been to cripple the country's economy, provoke abject poverty and despair in the people, and thus incite a popular rebellion against the government. Obama created a brief and superficial relaxation in the bilateral relations that led to the reestablishment of diplomatic ties and the introduction of a few-still timid-measures, that could have gradually brought about a normalization of relations. However, with the Donald Trump presidency, more than a regression, there has been an extraordinary worsening of aggression toward Cuba. Over 200 sanctions have been imposed on Cuba since Trump's inauguration, aimed at ruining the country. There is an embargo against fuel imports that has severely hurt the economy, public health, education, services, and the food supply of the Cuban people. An implacable tourism boycott was enforced; sales and donations of medications and medical equipment are blocked; stiff sanctions are applied to all financing schemes to assist the Island. Cuba cannot be sold any goods that contain more than 10% of U.S.-made components, regardless of the country where the goods are manufactured.

This policy naturally has a harsh impact, both directly and indirectly, on the development of public health in Cuba and on her efforts to exercise international solidarity, because doing so wreaks havoc on the domestic economy in general, and on the provisions of essential medical and pharmaceutical resources in particular. The United Nations has strongly opposed the blockage for decades to no avail, and at present, many countries, organizations, and personalities have called for an end to this criminal policy, at least during the pandemic, calls that the U.S. yet again has ignored. Even so, none of these obstacles has prevented Cuban cooperation.

At this point, with respect to this issue, a component of the smear campaigns deserves to be pointed out, which is the harassment by the U.S. of Cuba's health cooperation initiatives, precisely during the pandemic. Incredibly, the U.S. has been pressuring countries and threatening them with sanctions, brandishing completely false arguments to prevent their acceptance of Cuban aid.

Conclusions

The experience that Cuba has gained in the fight against COVID-19 proves that even a country faced by serious economic difficulties and subjected to an implacable embargo can confront a challenge of this pandemic's magnitude and suffer the least number of victims possible. This achievement has in essence been achieved thanks to longstanding policy decisions that have elevated humanity and social justice as Cuba's primordial objectives. The outcome has been that health care policies have been put in place, together with high-capacity infrastructure, and expert human resources have been trained of the highest professional, scientific, and technological caliber, who are prepared to serve the great majority of the population during intensive, prolonged outbreaks of epidemics or pandemics.

Moreover, the Cuban experience shows that when situations like this happen, there must be close, seamless coordination between all of the country's concerned institutions and organizations, the mass media and the people. The latter should be kept informed and advised on a daily basis regarding how to act in response to the unfolding events.

In sum, this pandemic teaches above all, though not exclusively, that health care must be a priority of national policymaking, and that in order for national policy to be effective, the State must have a strong foundation and place the needs of human beings first. It is indispensable to establish public, universal, and free—or accessibly priced—systems to serve the needs of the entire population. For this reason, far from constituting a solution, neoliberal policies are a serious obstacle or an impediment when problems such as the global spread of COVID-19 must be confronted. Neoliberal policies normally and irrationally place economic interests and mercantilism above the citizens' health.

On another note, Cuba's experience also suggests that countries ought to work to develop their own national medical-pharmaceutical industries; that they should not become totally subordinate to the modus operandi of large pharmaceutical consortia that profit from the business of medications. These consortia today are defining the research and development agendas based on the objectives of profit and revenues. Considerations of human well-being for the majority, above all in the countries of the Southern Hemisphere, are not central to their policies. Thus, if we are to avoid this dilemma and draw on the varied strengths of the countries of the South, it will be indispensable to achieve an integration that takes into account their complementary capabilities (Díaz-Canel, op.cit.). Leveraging national capacities through a solidary and rational approach to foreign policy, which has characterized the international conduct of Cuba and China, is therefore fundamental to combating epidemics, pandemics, and many other ills that affect the inhabitants of the planet.

Finally, Cuba's behavior in front of the present extreme situation also shows that it is impossible to isolate the health sector from the other national sectors, or from closely-related problems of an equal degree of seriousness as a pandemic. Intra-national and international inequality; hunger, poverty; deficient sanitation; wars of aggression that cause mass death and migration and force people to live in subhuman conditions and lead to the destruction of our natural environment—all of these phenomena either directly or indirectly impact on the capacity of countries and international organizations to face situations, such as the current one, that adversely affect the health of nations.

In synthesis, the problem is quite complex and we must confront it in a rational and solidary manner, over the foundation of globalized human fellowship, and setting aside political and ideological differences. Within this effort, Cuba and China have worked in a closely unified spirit, and the outcomes are there, for all to see.

VIII. Chile-China in Times of the Pandemic

Ricardo Santana Friedli[1]

"This [infection] curve will flatten outside the health care system, not inside it. The health care system is only here to cover the demand. This demand exists only if we are able to flatten the infection curve at the community level. We must be clear that we ourselves are the vehicle of contagion, and to the extent that we remain unaware of this fact, 60,000 vehicles will continue to drive out of the Metropolitan Region, forcing us to implement sanitary cordons to be in compliance with the regulations. Respect for the quarantine rules is fundamental. Channel 24 interview (Canal 24 Horas) with Dr. Héctor Sánchez, Director, Public Health Institute, Andrés Bello University (Instituto de Salud Pública de la Universidad Andrés Bello, UNAB).

May 19, 2020.

The Pandemic Begins

It was February 28 and from the presidential office in the Moneda Palace, Chilean president Sebastián Piñera made a call to his Chinese counterpart, President Xi Jinping, to express solidarity and offer Chile's help with the response to the ravages

---

1. Assistant Researcher CELC-UNAB.

of a little known virus. "The worst is over," Sebastián Piñera said, referring to the cases of infection in China and affirming the importance of cooperation in the fight against what was still categorized as an epidemic (GOB, 2020). The day before, a group with ties to China had met in a central location in the Santiago municipality of Providencia to record messages of support for the people of Wuhan, where the virus had emerged for the first time.

No one really knew what was coming; neither were people prepared for it in many countries.

Just two days before, after the call to the Chinese president, the first case of an infected person had been confirmed in Latin America. It was a Brazilian man from Sao Paulo who had traveled to Italy on February 9 had symptoms of fever, dry cough and sore throat. The virus would reach Chile two weeks later. Thus Chile ventured into the new international dynamic of a health crisis that was declared a pandemic the following week by the World Health Organization (Organización Mundial de la Salud, OMS).

Complicated weeks followed and oftentimes contradictions in the health measures and the statistics. In June 10, 2020 an article in the respected international journal "New Scientist" reported that Chile had the highest infection rate per million in South America, followed by Peru and Brazil, the U.S. and the U.K.

Chile lagged behind the other countries in the new "war for medical supplies". The international stage had already been contaminated by actions lacking any sense of cooperation or vision of a common strategy. "We are at war," announced French President Emmanuel Macron on March 16, after signing a decree allowing his government to requisition all necessary supplies for fighting the virus. The situation later led to tensions that triggered veritable threats and declarations that came and went between the Western countries. Such was the case of Spain and Italy, who accused France of confiscating four million masks ordered the Swedish company Mölnlycke from China.

The impasse was smoothed over after a flurry of diplomatic negotiations while the shipment was retained in French territory for 15 days. The consignment finally proceeded to its final destination after being disencumbered of half of the supplies. It happened again when Germany and France accused the U.S. of "theft" after U.S. officials at the Bangkok Airport confiscated medical supplies purchased in China by the European countries.

The shortage of masks and, later, ventilators, set off confrontations between neighboring countries and historical allies as though in the midst of a fight for survival. The virus went from being classed by several Western leaders early in the year as a "simple flu", to becoming a real national security threat. The events unfolding in Spain and Italy were observed from Chile as furores that no one wished to go through. Videos circulated on the web and social networks showing hospitals overcrowded with critically-ill patients, morgues filled with black body bags and medical teams on the verge of collapse. As all this was happening, the U.S. invoked a Korean War-era law to ban the export of domestically-produced masks, and instructed overseas U.S. companies to redirect their orders to their home country.

Chile-China Solidarity and Masks

The so-called "mask diplomacy" was already present in other countries and would soon emerge in Chile as well. Besides this, 2020 was already a year in which programs were being prepared to commemorate 50 years of uninterrupted diplomatic relations between Chile and China. The framework of interaction between the countries that was necessitated by the pandemic was defined by several "firsts": the first South American nation to establish diplomatic relations with China; the first Latin American country to recognize China as a market economy before the World Trade Organization (WTO); and the first nations to sign a free trade agreement (FTA) with the Asian power.

The objective data evidenced significant levels of commercial exchange and investment growth. Today China is the destination of 30% of total Chilean exports, according to 2019 figures (SUBREI, 2019). The success achieved by both parties enabled modernizing the FTA, which came into effect on March 1, 2019. Chile is also among the countries that have signed memoranda of understanding to join China's Belt and Road Initiative. Moreover, China has recently developed strategic investments in Chile that rose 167% in 2019, totaling USD $4.9 billion. China became the first to source of projects for InvestChile, the Chilean investment agency. These projects include the acquisition of 24% of SQM (lithium) by Tianqi Lithium Corporation and 100% of Chilquinta, an energy company (Zhu, 2020).

While Chile is not the only country in the region to receive Chinese investments, her favorable commercial and diplomatic relations with China became decisive for expediting the intricate process of medical acquisitions for the pandemic. The co-founder of Alibaba Foundation Jack Ma, tweeted, "One world, one battle!" as he made a donation through his Foundation of supplies to Africa, Asia, Europe and Latin America. Chile received 200,000 medical masks and 10 ventilators from Alibaba. However, these were not the last of the donations from China.

The e-commerce company Jing Dong donated 800,000 masks, 200,000 pairs of gloves and 15,000 protective gowns. Tianqi Lithium Corporation would later donate 100,000 masks and 20,000 N95 face masks. Likewise, the cities of Chengdu, Shenzhen and Ningbo delivered a total of 200,000 medical masks, while the government of Hubei Province, in commemoration of the canceled "Hubei Week" (an event to promote Hubei in the Chilean Region of Bio-Bio) made a donation of 10,000 disposable masks and 2,000 N95 masks (Castro, 2020).

Chinese ambassador to Chile Xu Bu commented that the donations to Chile from China totaled 2 million masks (of which over 20,000 were N95 masks), more than 200,000 pairs of medical gloves, 20,000 protective gowns, 20,000 infrared thermometers and 60 non-invasive ventilators (Bu, 2020). Thus, on April 21, when the pandemic was at its height in Chile, Health Minister Jaime Mañalich thanked the Chinese government and several Chinese associations for their donations.

Access to Medical Supplies

The interactions between Chile and China as a result of the pandemic coincide with China's growing international ascendancy and clear support for multilateralism. The masks and medical supplies have been China's demonstration of international solidarity and at the same time serve to strengthen ties with certain countries of interest. These developments have taken place amid her growing tensions with the U.S. At this time the U.S. shifted the focus of its anti-Beijing rhetoric from China the country to the Chinese Communist Party. There have been reactions, some stronger and others less so, from Europe and particularly from the U.K, stemming from disconcertment at the discovery of their strong interdependency vis-à-vis China and their need to fine-tune their policies with respect to the Asian power.

At the height of the global health crisis, China successfully and expeditiously responded to a test of its productive and management capability. In order to meet the demand of foreign markets overwhelmed by lockdowns and quarantines, China generated an overproduction of personal protection equipment (PPE) thanks to the reconversion capacity of the automotive, technological and textile industries, implemented in coordination with the central government. Thus China became these products' primary producer worldwide. Naturally some problems did arise when the equipment delivered by some companies, negotiated directly without the appropriate guarantees, did not match the purchasers' expectations or were lost in transport. Thus the United Nations warned that the incidence of fraud and theft of protective materials, even of COVID-19 tests, had risen, especially in Asia. And since the demand well exceeded the available supply, the requirement of advance payment has become common in exchange for priority access to the products (Noticias ONU, 2020).

Meanwhile, Chile was experiencing a rampant rise in infections in many parts of the country, with Santiago, the capital, registering the highest COVID-19 infection rate. The virus had reached Chile later and as a result the difficulties of obtaining the needed resources were now magnified as well. Suppliers were low on inventories, creating problems of access and compliance, as well as issues regarding standards and regulations that became bureaucratic bottlenecks in a situation of urgency.

Figure 1. Evolution of active COVID-19 cases in Chile as of July 2020 (By number of persons)

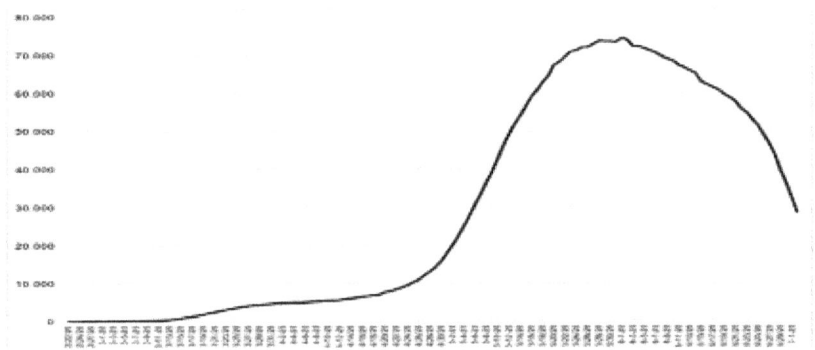

Source: Prepared by the authors based on statistical data from the Chile Ministry of Science, 2020.

Unlike other countries in the region, Chile has a strict public procurement system that requires payment for the goods or services contracted upon delivery or arrival at their requested destination. However, the factor of chaos in the international dynamic rendered the system obsolete for obtaining urgent medical supplies fabricated abroad.

The Chilean government was aware that the public system

would be hard-put to respond to the problem and turned to the Confederation of Production and Trade (*Confederación de la Producción y del Comercio*, CPC) to make use of the confederation's management capability. The CPC, headed by its president Juan Sutil, a Chilean agricultural businessman, began negotiations in China for the acquisition of the maximum permitted amounts of resources.

He received strong support from the Chilean Ambassador to China Luis Schmidt, also an agricultural entrepreneur and a longtime personal friend. At the peak of the pandemic, Chile was equipped with 1,229 ventilators available, 85% to 90% of which were being used to treat patients with common or stationary pathologies unrelated to the coronavirus. It was clear that prolonging this state of affairs would lead sooner or later to the collapse of Chile's entire health system. The CPC then sponsored the creation of a Private Emergency Fund to acquire ventilators and other medical supplies for public and private entities, that totaled more than $90 billion Chilean pesos (CPC, 2020).

The challenge for the business sector was to acquire as many provisions as possible in the shortest amount of time, while avoiding possible blockages or difficulties in the "war for medical supplies". To assist in this endeavor, the Chilean government provided Chilean Air Force (*Fuerza Aérea de Chile*, FACh) planes to prevent any possible requisitions and have the fewest layovers.

As Ambassador Schmidt later acknowledged in an interview, the risk of cargo requisitioning was high, therefore he took recourse to the Chilean Embassy in Beijing as a collection center, including the living and dining areas of the embassy residence. In spite of this, Ambassador Schmidt acknowledges that the Chinese authorities did authorize the supplies to leave the country and proceed to their destination, a demonstration of goodwill on the part of the Chinese government (Toro, 2020). Support was also forthcoming from local governments in identifying Chinese industries that complied with quality standards and offered fair prices.This was the Chinese authorities' way of showing that they wished to avoid the repetition of incidents such as those that occurred in Spain, with the sale of tests that were declared defective.

Chile depended on these efforts, because its official figures showed that the country was leading in infections and deaths in proportion to its population.

However, the fact was that within the region, reports were releasing doubtful information on coronavirus cases, whether because of deficient capacity of data gathering or political manipulation. In spite of methodological problems in the infection count (the number of deaths from the virus was modified up to three times), Chile has been able to perform a large number of tests in relation to the size of the population.

This is indicative of its real efforts to produce the most accurate figures possible.

Between the Pandemic and Extreme Scarcity

Notwithstanding the initial containment measures that the authorities put in place, the virus quickly traveled from the wealthier communities (early hotspots) to the poorest ones with fewer resources for withstanding the pandemic. The reality was revealed of thousands of Chileans who live in overcrowded, precarious conditions, and there was a revival of the social unrest of the historic demonstrations of October 2019, that an increase in Santiago subway fares had triggered. Twenty percent of Chileans live in a condition of multidimensional poverty. They suffer from deficiencies in education, health, work, social security, housing and in their general standard of living (PNUD, 2020).

Figure 2. Municipalities with the highest mortality in Santiago as of 29 June 2020

Comuna	Fallecidos
Puente Alto	341
La Florida	289
Maipú	229
Recoleta	227
San Bernardo	207
La Pintana	201
Peñalolén	192
Las Condes	180
Santiago	180
Cerro Navia	173
Independencia	165
Ñuñoa	161
Conchalí	152
Pudahuel	144
Renca	142
La Granja	142
Pedro Aguirre Cerda	140
El Bosque	129
Quinta Normal	116
Lo Espejo	112
Macul	103
San Ramón	102
Huechuraba	102
San Joaquín	100

Source: Prepared by the authors based on statistical data of the Epidemiological Report No. 29, Ministry of Health, 2020.

This is a determining socio-economic factor that explains why the largest numbers of COVID-19 deaths have been recorded in the capital's poorest municipalities (See Figure 2). Of the higher-income Santiago municipalities, just Las Condes chalks up 198 cases, and almost at the other end is Huechuraba with 102. The two municipalities have higher indices of overcrowding and informal employment—the informal labor force is estimated at 2.5 million nationwide—and a higher percentage of users of public transportation, who run a higher risk of contagion.

Fifty-six percent of the homes in Santiago have a surface area of less than 70 m2. The smallest-sized housing is in the municipalities of María Pinto (47.8 m2); San Pedro (48.37 m2), La Pintana (48 m2). In the more affluent sectors such as Lo Barnechea, houses have on average a surface area of 169.1 m2; in Vitacura 154.5 m2; and in Las Condes, 116.6 m2 (Molina, 2020). The municipalities of Independencia, San Bernardo, San Ramón and El Bosque have had the greatest difficulties in implementing the quarantine because they have large populations of unskilled workers and intensive users of public transport. It is one explanation for their high rates of fatalities. The Economic Commission for Latin America and the Caribbean (ECLAC) estimates that one repercussion of coronavirus in Chile will be a rise in poverty in 2020 of between 8.6% and 13.7%. On the other hand, in qualitative terms thousands of families live on what they earn from day to day, which renders them ineligible for the subsidies and benefits that have been forthcoming from the government.

Vaccines and Cooperation via Zoom

While in the first half of 2020 virus containment measures were put in place beyond China's borders and the competition began for medical supplies, in the second half of the year the so-called "vaccine war" gained visibility.

By mid-year the Chilean government was already in negotiations with three pharmaceutical companies: the UK's Oxford-Aztrazeca, and China's CanSino Biologics and Sinovac Biotech. The latter has already signed a cooperation agreement with the Catholic University of Chile (*Pontificia Universidad Católica de Chile*, PUC) for vaccine trials, the final experimental phase before rollout to the public (Yáñez, 2020). Note that this laboratory was the first to launch an H1N1 vaccine in the market against swine flu.

Indeed, the search for a vaccine has geopolitical dimensions, especially for China and the U.S. In June, three U.S. and four Chinese laboratories had announced that their vaccines were currently in Phase II of development (García, 2020). Trump is well aware that an announcement that a vaccine is in process of development in the U.S. could be a powerful message during a reelection campaign, with adverse voting forecasts because of how he has reacted to the coronavirus crisis. As for President Xi Jinping, he had announced before the 73rd World Health Assembly on May 18 that if China succeeded in finding a vaccine, it would be "for the use of all at an affordable price". He made the announcement in defense of the WHO's efforts to fight the pandemic, in complete contrast to Trump, who decided to withdraw the U.S. from the international body.

One thing is certain: the pandemic has revived the issue of

self-sufficiency in pharmaceutical production. In recent years, Europe and the U.S. have left the production of pharmaceuticals to other countries such as India, which has a monopoly over 50% of global vaccine output (Panday, 2020). This became a rude awakening for Europe, forced to scramble for a solution to a shortage of an essential drug produced abroad: paracetamol.

This international reality has been a recurring theme during the various debates in Chile on the state of public health and its future ramifications. The pandemic has exposed the necessity for information on other countries' experiences, especially China's, as the first country attacked by the virus, because of how she dealt with the pandemic. The keen interest in the results achieved by China through the lockdown and the measures to combat COVID-19 led to more webinars (online seminars) in Chile concerning the events in Asia.

China had much to share. Perhaps one of the first dialogs of this nature was held on March 27, entitled "The Chinese experience in the fight against the COVID-19 Pneumonia", with public health experts from Peking University. They gave live presentations on the measures implemented in Wuhan and what challenges had been tackled and had yet to be addressed, after living through two months of quarantine. The colloquium took place two days after the start of the first quarantine in Chile.

If there was a single takeaway from the online conference, the participants said it was the emphasis on social distancing as key to overcoming the pandemic. It was the experts' emphatic message. Dr. Yi Ning and Dr. Hong Ma were the main speakers at the event, organized by Tsinghua University Latin American Center (China) and several Chilean universities including Andrés Bello University (Universidad Andrés Bello, UNAB). Dr. Yi Ning is currently Executive Director of the Beijing Institute of Public Health Research. Dr. Hong Ma is the WHO Advisor for Asia-Pacific and also sits on China's expert panel on the control of COVID-19.

The event was a milestone in the successful partnership between Chile and China, the organizers said. "This was an excellent opportunity to connect with national and foreign universities and to learn from the Chinese doctors, who are weeks ahead of us in the control of this pandemic. It was a very significant learning experience," said Claudia Morales, Dean of UNAB School of Medicine. For Fabiola Novoa, Director of the Department of International Relations, UNAB, "Tsinghua University and UNAB have been strengthening their ties for ten years, with programs jointly promoted by the Center for Latin American Management of [Tsinghua] University and the UNAB Center for Latin American Studies on China (*Centro de Estudios Latinoaméricanos sobre China de la UNAB*, CELAC). "Representatives from both universities have maintained a fluid and productive dialog, which facilitated the meeting's organization. We can set distance aside and immerse ourselves in the questions and answers of a shared emergency."

According to Dr. Yi Ning, governments across the globe (the U.S., China, France, the U.K., Chile, etc.) are racing against time to develop a coronavirus vaccine. But until a cure for the disease is discovered, the doctor said, we must use a different approach to the problem: "The coronavirus spread much faster than we expected. We must take advantage of our certainties," he said. And what are those certainties? "If we know that the disease is highly contagious (more so than SARS of 2002), then the key is to isolate the patients who have the disease and protect the vulnerable population. In this way, we break the transmission chain." In other words: social distancing.

At the meeting the upheaval and disruption of the population' s normal lives as a result of rigorous confinement was discussed. Thus, above and beyond the clinical practice needed to stop the advance of the disease, one of the main aspects of maintaining control in cases of public health cases is the adequate application of a principle summarized by Dr. Hong Ma as Education Transparency: "Education for the population; transparency from the authorities." The academic insisted that the best way to attack a health emergency was through transparency on the part of the authorities to inspire the public's confidence in them. "Before introducing a massive health care measure, it is always advisable to carry out a trial to see if implementation is feasible," she said. Communication and the dissemination of protective measures must be done periodically, even if the messages are reiterative.

Another experience that led to direct dialog between China and Chile was the 10-day construction of a hospital in Wuhan to reinforce the medical care given to coronavirus patients. The dialog was held on June 10 and featured just one presentation, from Yu Di Hua, Chief Engineer of the General Contracting Company of China Construction Third Engineering Bureau (CCTEB) Co., Ltd. Nearly 100 professionals from Chile and China were in attendance for an in-depth discussion of the main technical challenges of the design and construction of the Huoshenshan Emergency Hospital. The event was organized by the Corporation of Technological Development of the Chilean Chamber of Construction (*Corporación de Desarrollo Tecnológico,* CDT; *Cámara Chilena de la Construcción,* CChC), in conjunction with the Chinese Council for the Promotion of Hubei Province International Trade (*Consejo Chino para la Promoción del Comercio Internacional de la Provincia de Hubei,* CCPIT-HUBEI), the China International Chamber of Commerce of Hubei Province in Chile (*la Cámara de Comercio Internacional de la Provincia de Hubei en Chile*) and the consulting firm Asia Reps, with the presence of several authorities of the sector.

The Chinese engineer spoke live, notwithstanding the time zone difference, and explained that the Huoshenshan Emergency

Hospital was built in ten work-intensive days on a surface area of nearly 50,000 square meters. The project itself has a built surface area of 33,940.76 square meters, and the hospital has a 1,000 bed capacity. Engineer Yu Di Hua explained said that the complex had "two buildings with hospitalization rooms and oxygen stations, with a negative pressure room and a wastewater treatment station." The hospital design is in the shape of an "L" to adapt to the site's topography and the layout of the medical units is like a "fishbone". He further explained, "It is a modular design and each fishbone is an independent medical unit. There are separate activity areas for the medical staff and the patients with traffic routes that comply with the hospital's functional design requirements."

After a presentation of video and graphics, other speakers participated, including Zhang Xiao Mei, President of the Hubei Province CCPIT, who placed special emphasis on the cooperation between the two countries. "Chile is the country farthest from China. At this extraordinary time, using a very different format than our usual one, we have overcome all the obstacles created by distance and by the virus. We have organized this exchange, which fully demonstrates that solidarity and cooperation are the most powerful weapons that the international community can use to defeat COVID-19," she indicated.

Luis Schmidt, Chilean Ambassador to China, sent greetings

and praised the high technical quality of both countries' construction industries.

"The world watched, amazed, as China built a hospital in less than 10 days. It is know-how and strategic skill worthy of being shared. Chile for her part has great know-how in construction. Living in one of the most seismic countries in the world, Chileans have the ability to build great engineering works that are recognized worldwide," he said.

A Post-Pandemic Look

Chile is especially focusing on a future permanent dialog between Chinese and Chilean experts in different areas. A project is being promoted for the installation of an optical fiber cable that will join the Chilean coast to Southeast Asia. The project is congruent with Chile's vision of China's Belt and Road Initiative, a vision whose scope goes beyond merely two pathways, one land-based and the other maritime. The flight routes achieved by 20th century advances should be added as well. The digital road will finally eliminate the problem of physical distance from China-instead our attention will focus much more on shared interests and visions in a global environment.

As the concrete expression of the diplomacy that is possible to sustain via the digital route, the high-level video conference convened on June 19 by the Minister of Foreign Affairs of the

People's Republic of China, Wang Yi, promoted closer united action against COVID-19 and encouraged economic recovery through cooperation among the partners of the Belt and Road Initiative. Chile is an associated country of the Initiative and Minister Teodoro Ribera and Assistant Secretary of International Economic Relations Rodrigo Yañez were participants at the meeting. Minister Ribera emphasized the importance of multidimensional international cooperation to overcome the economic crisis of COVID-19. "In the current international context, the commitment of all countries to support an open trading system that is non-discriminatory and based on transparent norms is especially important. These are fundamental conditions to successfully recover from this global economic crisis," stressed the Chilean minister.

He also urged the countries present "to work together at this critical time and to refrain from introducing measures that restrict trade and may constitute unnecessary barriers to it". Minister Ribera encouraged his audience "to guarantee trade flows in order to achieve a successful and expeditious economic and commercial recovery, essential conditions to ensure the subsistence of our citizens." He also called for more international cooperation and coordination, in order to build consensus around and achieve the Sustainable Development Goals (SDA) of Agenda 2030. Specifically, referring to the ties between Chile and China, Minister Ribera also emphasized the signing by both countries last April of a joint declaration, within the framework of the free trade agreement (FTA), pledging to strengthen cooperation and combat COVID-19. In it the countries recognized the importance of supporting the free flow of goods and services, connectivity and keeping supply chains open to achieve sustainable economic growth (SUBREI, June 2020). The final paragraph defined shared criteria with a comprehensive reach in the current state of international affairs:

"Both parties will closely collaborate to better implement the bilateral FTA, which plays an important role in facilitating the free flow of goods and services, supporting the integrity of global supply chains, mitigating the impacts of the pandemic on bilateral trade and investment, and contributing to more sustainable economic growth after the crisis. The two countries will adopt the necessary measures to ensure the continuous flow of vital medical supplies and equipment, critical agricultural products and other cross-border goods and services required to protect the health of their citizens. They will work together to assist vulnerable developing countries and less-developed nations. Both countries assume a commitment to support the Multilateral Trade System and agree that emergency measures for tackling COVID-19 must be concrete, transparent and temporary, and should also be compatible with the rules established by the WTO."

The statement was a concrete demonstration of how the bridges built between Chile and China over the years are the relevant framework for addressing the effects of the pandemic and the post-pandemic challenges that will arise.

IX. A New Crisis Piled Over Old Crises: COVID-19 in Bolivia and Latin America

Nicole Jordán Prudencio[1]

Introduction

Diseases have always been part of the human experience; however, a combination of global trends, including...extreme weather, has heightened the risk.... [T]here is a very real threat that a pandemic may be unleashed by a highly lethal and contagious respiratory pathogen, capable of killing between 50 and 80 million people and wiping out around 5% of the world economy. A global pandemic of such a magnitude would be catastrophic, creating widespread havoc, instability, and insecurity. The world is not prepared. (Dr. Brundtland, G. & Sy, E., GPMB, 2019, p. 6)

Years ago, numerous scientific studies were already sounding the alert of the elevated risk of a pandemic similar to the current one (Chenget al., 2007; Menachery, V. et al., 2015; National Academy of Medicine, 2016). However, the warnings

1. Political Scientist, professor at the Universidad Católica Boliviana; Sustainable Development Projects Coordinator, FES-Bolivia.

did not have the impact that was necessary to prevent an outbreak or mitigate its devastating consequences. On one hand, the needed restrictions and controls to prevent the sale of wild animals for human consumption were not imposed (or, failing this, the implementation of appropriate bio-safety measures), even when the potential danger to health of this type of trade has long been known.[2] On the other hand, according to the Global Health Security Index (known as the GHS Index)[3] first published in 2019, no health system in the world has been sufficiently prepared to face such a scenario. This last point elucidates the serious difficulties that all the countries have had to grapple with (and continue to do) in managing the global health crisis triggered by the coronavirus (COVID-19).

Together with Africa, Latin America has been one of the hardest-hit regions, primarily due to a series of economic, health-related, social, and political factors, among them: low levels of economic growth in the period prior to the pandemic's advent, limited tax revenue collection and rising central government public debt. These factors were serious constraints for public

2. More than 70% of human diseases come from wild animals. While some countries have begun to ban markets that sell wild game, the danger is that instead of doing away with the markets, such bans will only force them to migrate underground to illegal and digital markets.

3. The Global Health Security Index is a project by the Johns Hopkins University Health Security Center in conjunction with The Economist Intelligence Unit. It is the first comprehensive health security tool to look at 195 countries around the world and evaluate their capacity to prevent and mitigate epidemics and pandemics.

spending, which is essential to mitigate the negative effects of the pandemic (ECLAC, 2020). There was allocation of resources to the public health systems, and to innovation, research, and development in science and technology, there were high rates of poverty and inequality, with the gains made showing a regressive trend beginning in 2015 (CEPAL, 2018). In sum, many were left facing a veritable dilemma: caught between the fear of dying from COVID-19, or dying from hunger.

Bolivia straddles this set of circumstances, having recently come under the international spotlight following the political and social crisis that was triggered by the October 2019 presidential elections. The electoral process was marred by serious irregularities and fraud that undermined the credibility and integrity of the vote. Several episodes ensued of social conflict throughout the country that culminated in the resignation and self-exile of then-President Evo Morales, and the disruption of the social fabric. Thus the multi-dimensional crisis that is the coronavirus pandemic (COVID-19) is piled on top of the already-profound political and social crisis previously installed in Bolivia. And as if this were not enough, the pandemic was the add-on to an economic slowdown exacerbated, initially, by the stoppage of the economy during the unrest of 2019 and, subsequently, by the economic collapse as a result of the lockdown measures put in place around the world.

All of these factors as a whole render even more complex

the enormous challenges both and future and demands that we reflect on how to manage these multiple challenges and turn them into opportunities for spurring the changes needed in Bolivia and in other countries of the region. Given the limitations of space and time, all aspects of the global crisis cannot be addressed in a single document; therefore this article will focus on the heart of it all: health care.

Accordingly, this document will provide a brief overview of the pre-pandemic status of the health care system in Bolivia compared to that of the other health care systems of 18 selected Latin American countries.[4] Its primary objective is to draw lessons that will enable opening up the public debate on those aspects that must be targeted for improvement. These will include, on one hand, the capacities and present condition of the health systems and, on the other, the Bolivian and other Latin American governments' readiness and response strategies for coping with future health emergencies. The first part of this proposal is to shed light on the pre-existing structural vulnerabilities in Bolivia, and that are also common across the region. Second, to explore how Bolivia and the region have performed with respect to the large-scale testing needed for

4. The selected Latin American countries aside from Bolivia are: Argentina, Brazil, Chile, Colombia, Costa Rica, Ecuador, El Salvador, Guatemala, Haiti, Honduras, Mexico, Nicaragua, Panama, Paraguay, Peru, Dominican Republic, Uruguay and Venezuela. From this point on, when we refer to the region or to the Latin American countries, please keep in mind that we mean the countries selected for this analysis.

the detection of coronavirus (COVID-19). Third, to perform a comparative analysis of some of these same factors vis-à-vis China, to identify similarities and differences. Finally, to try and draw the most outstanding lessons that are applicable to Bolivia and the rest of the countries under analysis, and suggest how China can adopt a more proactive role in the actions of cooperation for development in Latin America, to contribute in greater measure to the objective set out in this document.

Ready or Not... Here Comes Coronavirus!

Before the virus reached Latin America, and after the world witnessed how health care systems far better prepared for it were overwhelmed, as in Italy and in Spain, it became evident that neither the public nor private health care systems in Bolivia were prepared to deal with the impact of the pandemic. Bolivia was in position number 102 out of 195 countries in the GHS index (Johns Hopkins University, 2019).[5] As seen in Table 1, according to the Index the Latin American countries less prepared than Bolivia for facing the pandemic (of the other 18 included in this analysis) are Guatemala, Haiti, Honduras, and Venezuela (not considering Paraguay, which scored just one point less than Bolivia). This vision aligns with the June

5. The higher positioned a country is in the ranking, the better prepared it is in terms of health security. The optimal score is 100.

2020 Report of the World Health Organization (WHO, 2020) on the status of countries with respect to strategic readiness and response capacity for coping with the coronavirus (COVID-19). The report lists Bolivia as a country with limited capacity (Level 2 out of 5).

Table 1. Global Health Security Index 2019 Applied to Selected Countries in Latin America

País	Prevención (sobre 100)	Detección Temprana (sobre 100)	Respuesta Rápida y Mitigación (sobre 100)	Sistema de Salud (sobre 100)	Normas (sobre 100)	Entorno de Riesgo (sobre 100)	Puntaje Promedio (sobre 100)	Ranking (de 195 países)
Argentina	41.4	74.9	50.6	54.9	68.8	60.0	58.6	25
Bolivia	44.0	33.1	29.2	14.9	48.5	50.9	35.8	102
Brasil	59.2	82.4	67.1	45.0	41.9	56.2	59.7	22
Chile	56.2	72.7	60.2	39.3	51.5	70.1	58.3	27
Colombia	37.2	41.7	43.5	34.3	60.1	51.0	44.2	65
Costa Rica	44.2	56.0	36.6	24.8	43.1	71.7	45.1	62
Ecuador	53.9	71.2	39.5	35.2	43.5	57.1	50.1	45
El Salvador	22.1	73.9	42.1	25.2	50.5	48.0	44.2	65
Guatemala	21.2	50.0	25.0	11.4	42.2	49.1	32.7	125
Haití	31.5	48.3	21.1	10.6	48.4	28.9	31.5	138
Honduras	21.6	27.7	26.5	12.0	41.8	39.5	27.6	156
México	45.5	71.2	50.8	46.9	73.9	57.0	57.6	23
Nicaragua	41.7	39.9	39.2	45.9	51.8	41.0	43.1	73
Panamá	40.5	44.6	46.4	35.1	35.3	63.8	43.7	68
Paraguay	39.5	34.6	26.8	28.2	35.3	55.9	35.7	103
Perú	43.2	38.3	51.7	45.0	63.0	57.7	49.2	49
Rep. Dominicana	30.5	37.1	47.3	16.1	43.5	59.3	38.3	91
Uruguay	44.0	33.5	41.3	24.1	39.3	74.8	41.3	81
Venezuela	23.5	8.7	19.7	12.9	42.2	38.2	23.0	176

Source: Created by the author based on country profiles in the Johns Hopkins 2019 University Global Health Security Index.
Notes: (A) Only 19 of the total 33 countries in Latin America were considered. These 19 are the countries listed in the Index. (B) The categories explored in the index are: 1) Prevention of the emergence or release of pathogens; 2) early detection and reporting of epidemics with potential for becoming of international concern; 3) rapid response to and mitigation of the spread of an epidemic; 4) adequate and robust health system to treat the sick and protect health workers; 5) compliance with international standards, including adherence to global norms, commitment to improving national capacity and financing plans to address gaps; 6) risk environment and vulnerability of the country to biological threats. (C) Countries are highlighted that scored and ranked lower than Bolivia.

Although Bolivia's average score in the 2019 GHS Index was 35.8 out of 100 (see Table 1)–not far from the scores of other countries–, its score for specifically measuring the capacity of clinics, hospitals, and community health centers was barely 3.6 out of 100, ranking Bolivia above just three countries: Guatemala, Honduras, and Haiti (See Table 2). If other crucial indicators are considered for measuring country capacity to face a pandemic, such as having a contingency plan in place to tackle a national health emergency or having a minimum number of epidemiologists and epidemiology training programs, it is chilling to realize that Bolivia scored 0 for both of these indicators.

Table 2. Health System Capacity for Detection, Response, and Management of the Selected Latin American Countries for Coping with a Pandemic Based on 5 Indicators of the 2019 GHS Index

PAÍS	SISTEMAS DE LABORATORIO	SISTEMAS DE VIGILANCIA EPIDEMIOLÓGICA	EPIDEMIOLOGÍA (FUERZA LABORAL Y PROGRAMAS DE CAPACITACIÓN)	PLAN ANTE EMERGENCIA NACIONAL DE SALUD	CAPACIDAD EN CENTROS DE SALUD	PROMEDIO SOBRE 100
Argentina	83,3	70	50	50	46	59,86
Bolivia	66,7	58,3	0	0	3,6	25,72
Brasil	100	81,7	50	87,5	55,6	74,96
Chile	83,3	61,7	50	37,5	6,1	47,72
Colombia	66,7	43,3	50	0	7,4	33,48
Costa Rica	83,3	56,7	75	0	5,1	44,02
Ecuador	83,3	80	25	37,5	32,9	51,74
El Salvador	50	75	75	25	22,6	49,52
Guatemala	66,7	26,7	100	0	3,5	39,38
Haití	50	36,7	100	0	1,6	37,66
Honduras	33,3	0	75	12,5	2,8	24,72
México	83,3	80	25	25	51,2	52,9
Nicaragua	66,7	60	25	0	46,2	39,58
Panamá	50	46,7	75	75	51	59,54
Paraguay	50	56,7	25	0	5,8	27,5
Perú	33,3	86,7	25	87,5	6,3	47,76
Rep. Dominicana	33,3	35	75	50	7	40,06
Uruguay	33,3	45	50	37,5	17,7	36,7
Venezuela	33,3	0	0	0	6,4	7,94

Source: Created by the author based on country profiles in the Johns Hopkins 2019 University Global Health Security Index. Notes: (a) Only 19 Latin American countries are included. (b) Countries are highlighted whose average scores are lower than Bolivia's.

While it is true that Bolivia is not alone in the region in having no emergency plan, it is only Bolivia and Venezuela that have no policies to ensure the creation of a specialized labor force and the putting in place of training programs in epidemiology (See Table 2). The reasons for the two countries' lack of such policies are quite divergent and defy comparison- Bolivia has seen a decade of sustained economic growth while Venezuela has been submerged in an unprecedented humanitarian crisis for years.

This leads to the question: has public health been a priority for Bolivia? One possible approach to an answer would be to measure the percentage of public spending that the country has allocated to health care in recent years, and compare it to those of other countries in the region and beyond. As shown in Figure 1, as of 2017 very few Latin American countries earmarked more than 5% of GDP to spending on public health administration. Based on World Bank data, average allocation to health in 2017 for Latin America and the Caribbean was 4.2%, considerably lower than the health investment for the same time period in the European Union (7.42%) or North America (U.S., 8.56% and Canada, 7.79%).

While these are interesting figures, they should be seen in the context of each country's total population, as the variable that establishes the sufficiency or deficiency of the percentage allocated to health. Cross-referencing the information makes it possible to establish that, although Bolivia was slightly above the Latin American average in terms of public spending on health care (Figure 1), it still lagged behind Paraguay, Nicaragua, El Salvador, Costa Rica, Panama, and Uruguay. These countries earmark a similar percentage of GDP to health, but their total populations are approximately half or a third of Bolivia's (Figure 2).

The gap becomes even more glaring upon comparing the figures for public spending on health per capita. At US$ 150.90

in 2017, Bolivia is far behind the Latin American average (US$ 343.82, considering only the countries of the region included in this study), and only ranks higher than Nicaragua, Guatemala, Honduras, Haiti, and Venezuela (WHO, 2020c).

Figure 1. Public Spending on Health in Selected Latin American Countries, 2017 (% of GDP)

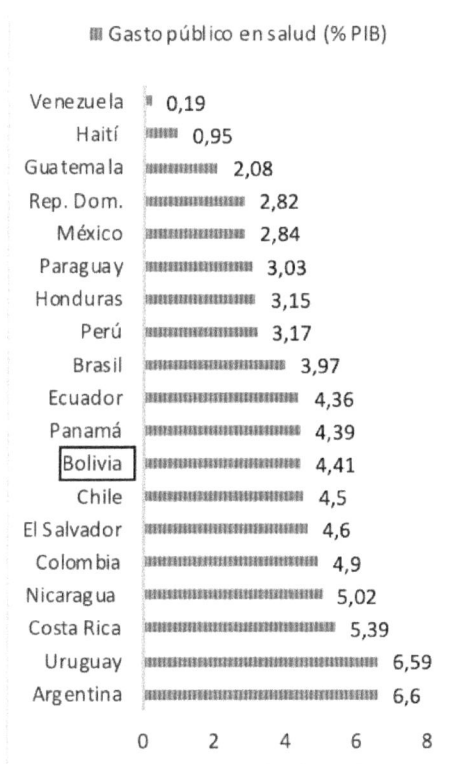

▥ Gasto público en salud (% PIB)

Country	% PIB
Venezuela	0,19
Haití	0,95
Guatemala	2,08
Rep. Dom.	2,82
México	2,84
Paraguay	3,03
Honduras	3,15
Perú	3,17
Brasil	3,97
Ecuador	4,36
Panamá	4,39
Bolivia	4,41
Chile	4,5
El Salvador	4,6
Colombia	4,9
Nicaragua	5,02
Costa Rica	5,39
Uruguay	6,59
Argentina	6,6

Source: Created by the author based on World Bank data and Global Health Spending information from the WHO, 2017.
Note: (a) GGHE-D%GDP (measure), (b) Only the 19 countries in Latin America are considered.

Figure 2. Total Population in Selected Countries of Latin America, 2018 (In Millions)

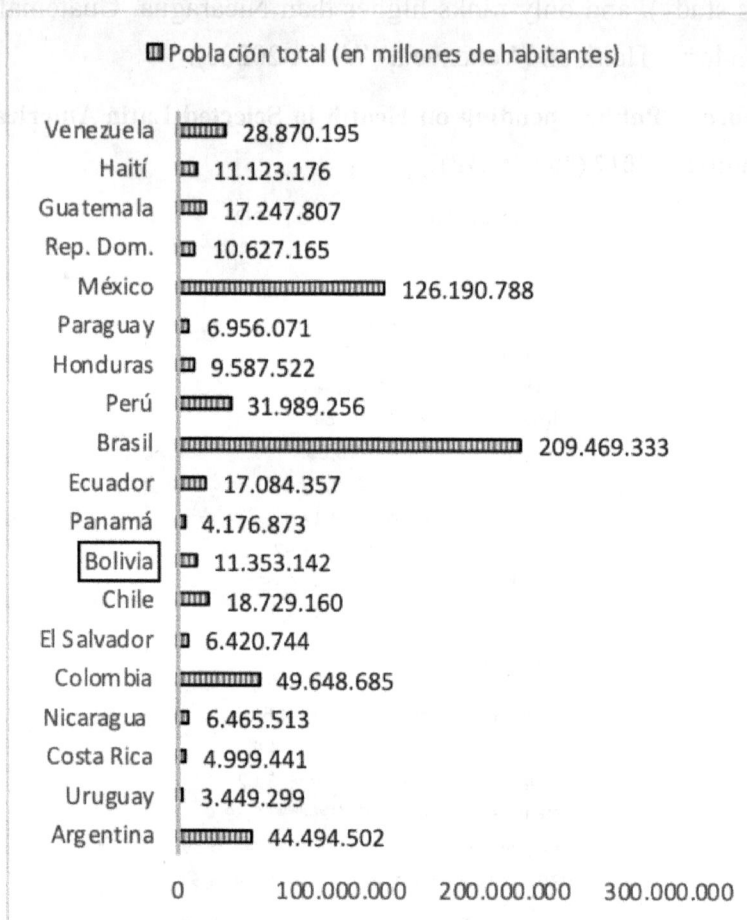

Población total (en millones de habitantes)

Venezuela	28.870.195
Haití	11.123.176
Guatemala	17.247.807
Rep. Dom.	10.627.165
México	126.190.788
Paraguay	6.956.071
Honduras	9.587.522
Perú	31.989.256
Brasil	209.469.333
Ecuador	17.084.357
Panamá	4.176.873
Bolivia	11.353.142
Chile	18.729.160
El Salvador	6.420.744
Colombia	49.648.685
Nicaragua	6.465.513
Costa Rica	4.999.441
Uruguay	3.449.299
Argentina	44.494.502

Source: Created by the author based on World Bank data, 2018. Note: Only 19 Latin America countries are considered.

Allocation of public money to health is not necessarily proportional to the size of the economies, but is rather directly tied to a vision of health as a public good, which leads to the notion that it ought to be prioritized above other spending and investment for governments. This, in contrast with other visions that are more oriented toward the privatization of health care services. This is evidently the case of Brazil, which allocates very few public resources to health care, despite its population density which is exponentially higher than that of the rest of Latin America. The same can be said of the Asian giant, China, with a total population of around 1.4 billion people in 2018, that spent 2.9% of its GDP to public health spending, or US$ 249.80 per capita in 2017, according to statistics for these years from the World Bank and WHO.

Specifically, with respect to health center capacity in terms of human resources and essential facilities, there is an enormous gap between Bolivia and the rest of the region. Just before the pandemic reached Latin America, Bolivia was already ranked the third country with the least number of doctors, 47.6 on average per 100,000 inhabitants, ranking only higher than Honduras and Haiti, far behind Argentina (390.7) and Uruguay (373.6), and lagging significantly behind Ecuador (166.5) and Venezuela (192.5). Another critical factor to consider is the number of hospital beds per 100,000 people. Bolivia has 110 hospital beds for every 100,000 Bolivians, just slightly more than Nicaragua,

Venezuela, Haiti, Honduras, and Guatemala.

Add to this outlook the dearth of specialists and Intensive Care Units (ICUs) to attend to critical care patients, and the scenario becomes that much more complex for Latin America, and in particular for Bolivia.

By way of example, the WHO stipulates that there should be, on average, one ICU bed for every 10,000 persons. However, as of April 4, 2020, Bolivia had just 430 ICU beds in the entire health care system, public and private, when a minimum of 1,163 units would be needed, or nearly thrice as many; just 210 specialists when 600 were needed for a population of approximately 11,633,000 people, according to the INE projection for 2020 (Alanoca, 2020; Chuquimia, 2020; La Prensa Digital, 2020). In contrast, as of the same date Paraguay had 775 ICU beds (public and private sector) and 178 ICU specialists (UltimaHora, 2020). This is a difference of nearly twice as many more ICU beds in Paraguay for a population nearly 50% smaller than that of Bolivia.

ICU wards in Bolivia are not prepared to provide care to critical COVID-19 patients due to a deficit of human resources, infrastructure, equipment, supplies, and drugs, but also primarily due to a lack of personal protection needed for health workers to stay safe while coping with this health crisis (Salvatierra et al., 2020).

Given the state of the health care system, it is understandable that strict lockdown measures have been in place since the health emergency began in Bolivia, because an out-of-control rise in the number of cases in Brazil could quickly lead to the collapse of the system nationwide, a scenario that unfortunately does not seem very far off. A clear example is Beni, the Department with the second-highest number of confirmed COVID-19 cases (4,275 people as of July 5, 2020), according to the official government website Bolivia Segura, and whose health system is one of the most precarious in the country. The epicenter of the pandemic is still in the Department of Santa Cruz, with 21,752 confirmed cases (Ibid.), however the case of Beni is emblematic because at the moment when number of cases spiked in the department, it only had three ICU specialists, in a population of nearly half a million people.[6] The rapid rise of infections in the department, added to the lack of specialists and support staff, led to a situation in which personnel with little training in acute care had to work day and night, despite the fact that many of them had caught the disease themselves, to prevent people from dying due to lack of care (Pérez, 2020; UNITEL, 2020). Generally speaking, the lack of specialized staff, the inadequate hospital infrastructure,[7] shortages of biosafety equipment for the

6. Interview with Jorge Gómez, Director, Beni Department Health Service (SEDES). conducted on May 19, 2020 by UNITEL Bolivia.

7. More than 90% of health care facilities in Bolivia are primary care facilities, thus they do not have the minimal conditions needed to treat critical care patients (Salvatierra et al., 2020).

personal protection for health workers, rea-gents for COVID-19 testing, absence of a national crisis management plan, and the overworking of the few labs with the capacity to carry out diagnostic testing due to the high demand, among a myriad of other problems, brought the country to the edge, which is even more daunting considering that Bolivia was already in a rather inauspicious position for confronting a health emergency of this nature.

After the first reports of people dying in their homes from lack of medical care, or on the streets of various cities and even in the lobbies of some medical centers, fears arose that we could be entering a critical phase of national systemic collapse.

Absent the equipment, absent the infrastructure, and absent the ICU specialists, we will be unable to do anything. Acute patients need 24-hour ventilator care and if they do not receive medication their lives will be in danger. The entire health care system is already collapsing and still the number of cases is on the rise. "What will happen to the patients who need intensive care? There are difficult days ahead" (Interview with Adrián Ávila, President, Bolivia Intensive Care Society, La Prensa Digital, 2020).

The Reality of Bolivia and Latin America: A Blind Struggle for Survival

As mentioned earlier, the 2019 GHS Index indicates that, of

the 195 countries assessed, only 13 are classed in the category of best-prepared to confront a pandemic, and not one of them is Latin American. The U.S. heads the list with a score of 83.5 out of 100, while China comes in at just 48.2 (Johns Hopkins University, 2019). Curiously, despite these high levels of preparedness, it quickly became clear that the pandemic was not optimally managed in the U.S. In fact, several health care systems, including that of New York, collapsed, something that heretofore was unthinkable. To date (July 5, 2020), the U.S. continues to be the country with the highest number of cases confirmed and deaths from COVID-19 worldwide. Confirmed cases total 2,879,830 and the death toll, 129,912, although these figures are also a reflection of the U.S. Being the country that conducts the most tests per day per thousand inhabitants (Our World in Data, 2020).

China's figures are much lower in comparison: 84,868 confirmed cases and 4,641 deaths to date, despite having been the pandemic's ground zero (Johns Hopkins University, 2020). Although previous comparisons showed that China was lagging behind in terms of public spending on health, or specific capabilities tied to the indicators of the 2019 GHS Index, in mass testing China has proven to be a true global power, having tested a total of 9.9 million people in Wuhan alone as of June 1, 2020, according to the city authorities.[8] In other words, more than the

8. There is no independent source available to confirm these data (Reality Check Team, 2020).

average number of tests performed in Latin America.

These numbers show that, while readiness and capabilities are key for dealing with a situation such as the current one, crisis management and timely responses can also make all the difference in the number of lives saved. Accordingly, one recommendation made by several international agencies that should be part of any plan before or during the lifting of lockdowns in countries, whose efficaciousness is proven regardless of the type of society it is applied in, is widespread, frequent testing. This is because it is impossible to fight a pandemic when you do not know who has caught the disease (OECD, 2020; Nature, 2020).

In contrast to the conditions in China or the U.S., the main problem in most of the Latin American countries is that they have had neither the capacity nor the resources to conduct the mass testing required for early, timely diagnosis that saves lives and slows the spread of the disease.

The analysis of the statistics of confirmed COVID-19 cases and testing performed suggests that, on average, the countries with the most confirmed cases are precisely those that perform the most lab tests. Since none of the Latin American countries are performing enough tests per day, and given that a considerable number of carriers may be asymptomatic, it is impossible to be certain what the real figures are of the number of people infected with COVID-19 in the region. Thus it is that the countries find themselves in a blind struggle against an enemy that surely is more powerful than initially thought.

A review of the figures and graphs points to Paraguay as being one of the most interesting cases. Paraguay has recently been praised for its successful management of the crisis, compared to other countries in the region that had appeared to be better prepared. Its success has sparked many questions, such as: How did a country like Paraguay with baseline constraints on par with those of Bolivia in terms of its precarious health care system, achieve such different outcomes with respect to the numbers of infected, recovered and deaths from COVID-19?

Paraguay and Bolivia are both landlocked countries in a situation of internationally isolation, and this may have contributed to reducing the spread of the virus to some extent. Likewise, as per the 2019 GHS Index and the WHO, Paraguay's health system capacity is comparable to that of Bolivia. However, as of June 27, 2020 Paraguay had recorded a total of 1,711 confirmed cases, 1,013 recovered cases, and 15 deaths, compared to Bolivia's 29,423 confirmed cases, 7,736 recovered cases, and 934 deaths from COVID-19, within the same time period (See Figures 4, 6 and 7). Because Paraguay has done more testing than Bolivia within the same time window, despite having a much smaller population, it is easy to rule out the hypothesis that the difference in the numbers may be due to testing less people. One fundamental factor that sets Paraguay apart would seem to be population density. The country's total population is very small compared to other countries in the region. That is why the Paraguayan health system appears similar to that of Bolivia, but in reality has greater capacity. For example, Paraguay has approximately three times as many doctors per 100,000 persons as does Bolivia (See Figures 2 and 3). This criterion would partially explain why it is that, despite the similarities between the two countries, Paraguay has been able to better contain the spread of the virus and offer better care to acute patients, thus greatly reducing the number of people who have died and raising the recovery rate.

Something else that has been decisive for the successful management of the crisis throughout the region are the decisions made and actions taken by central governments in coordination with local governments, as well as their communication strategies, and, finally, the approval level or willingness of their societies to cooperate or respond positively to how the crisis was managed. For these reasons, while there are various international recommendations that can be replicated because of to their widespread positive effects, such as travel protocols, social distancing, hygiene measures and food-handling procedures, among many others, it is imperative that each country evaluate the extent to which said guidelines can be effectively implemented in each national context. Returning to the initial point, Latin America is in the midst of a particularly fragile economic situation, given the context described in detail at the beginning of this writing. This is why the economic mea-sures undertaken by the Bolivian government to mitigate the impact of the crisis in the population[9] have been insufficient or have been undermined by logistical, communicational, and political problems, leading many sectors to lobby to reopen the economy, and many people to breach the quarantines, especially those who work in the subsistence economy.

Added to this is a difficult prior political and social situation, the string of conflicts that spread throughout the region in 2019 whose common denominator was social unrest. In Bolivia's case the situation is even more delicate, because the interim government does not enjoy the majority support of the Plurinational Legislative Assembly, it does not have the legitimacy it needs to be able to negotiate such a complex crisis, and it is unable to make long-term decisions to mitigate its impacts. Indeed, as though the foregoing did not already translate into a general outlook for Bolivia of instability and a problematic governability, the corruption scandals that have emerged around medical supply purchases have eroded popular confidence in the government's management of the crisis (Miranda, 2020) and the electoral process is plagued by political and social polarization.

9. These measures include bonuses, deferred bank loan payments, discounts for utility charges (power, water, gas), bans on the suspension of these basic services and of Internet for the duration of strict lockdowns, etc.

Finally, from a more sociological and anthropological point of view, it is evident that social and cultural practices inherent to Latin American countries can make it difficult for social distancing and other pandemic-related rules to be observed with the same degree of adherence as in other societies.

In Bolivia, for example, it is important to bear in mind that self-medicating is a very common practice society. This is due first of all to the fact that most people only go to the doctor when they have symptoms that are more serious than a cold.

Second, the continuing importance of traditional medicine for wide sectors of the population. Third, besides the above-mentioned factors, restrictions on the purchase of over-the-counter pharmaceuticals are much weaker than in other countries. If one adds to this scenario the worldwide uncertainty and discrepancies around the issue of what the best way is to treat COVID-19 patients, and, on the other, the abundant and ubiquitous misinformation circulating on social media, and the widespread fears of a population that feels unprotected by a fragile and overwhelmed health care system, then clearly there is a high risk of people ingesting toxic products, or improper doses of drugs or even overdosing on certain medicines. All of this could end up in other types of complications that have already become visible in COVID-19 patients in Bolivia (Ministerio de Salud, 2020b).

How to Foster "Change by Design and not by Disaster" in the Midst of a Catastrophe?

Pre-existing precariousness, as well as the fault lines exposed by the pandemic, clearly point to the high degree of vulnerability that ails not just Bolivian, but all Latin American societies, with respect to social protection in the sphere of health care. It is evident that a change is required in government spending priorities. Policies must be geared more toward strengthening and improving health care services and systems overall. While it may seem that at this late hour fostering "change by design and not by catastrophe", as Álvaro Cálix[10] has asserted, is no longer possible, we can still extract valuable lessons that can contribute to health systems that are more resilient and strategic policies for managing the crisis.

That said, some of the main conclusions of this document point at the following:

• In Bolivia, as in many of the Latin American countries analyzed here, the health crisis was piled on top of pre-existing economic, political, and social crises, rendering the situation even more complex.

• Most health care systems in Latin America were unprepared to deal with health emergencies, primarily due to

10. Paraphrasing of a statement by Álvaro Cálix during his presentation at a virtual regional meeting in April 2020 of the Social-Ecological Transformation Project, sponsored by the Friedrich Ebert Foundation.

lack of supplies, infrastructure, equipment and specialists, not to mention the absence of policies and emergency plans. Although these problems are common to all the countries of the region, as far as Bolivia is concerned, the scenario is even worse given the great gaps between her and her Latin American peers.

• Suboptimal administration of COVID-19 tests in Bolivia, as well as in most other Latin American countries, greatly limits Bolivia's ability to manage the spread of COVID-19 and provide good care to the sick population.

• The lack of public investment in health is common across the region, with the exception of a few countries. This is due to budgetary constraints, but also to different approaches to health. The pandemic makes it pressing for Latin American governments to rethink their priorities and make health, in practice, a basic human right and common good. To achieve this there will need to be not just better access and coverage, but also improved service quality.

Regarding this last point, although unlike many countries in the region Bolivia does have a Universal Healthcare System (*Sistema Universal de Salud*, SUS), which guarantees "universal, equitable, timely and free access" (Ministerio de Salud, 2020c) to Bolivians who do not have health insurance, the implementation of the SUS has not been as successful as initially anticipated. Given the high percentage of informal workers in Bolivia, the expansion of health coverage is an imperative requiring a deepened commitment. However, to date, the precarity of the health services leaves recipients dissatisfied. What then would be the the point of expanding coverage of a service that does not even meet the minimum requirements for care of its pacients?

Thus, there is a need not only to expand coverage but also to improve the quality of health care services in Bolivia. To do so, resources will have to be managed intelligently and efficiently so as to have a sustainable system over time, with support from international cooperation.

China and her Strategic Ties to the Region

Throughout the global health crisis, China has assumed a central role in international cooperation and humanitarian aid by sending experts, supplies and medical equipment in high demand when many countries are straining to extend any sort of assistance because they too are struggling with their own national crises. Thus, between April and March 2020, more than 100 countries across the globe, Bolivia included, received donations from private Chinese enterprises as well as from the government of the People's Republic of China (Los Tiempos, 2020; Ministerio de Salud, 2020a; Mulakala and Hongbo, 2020).

And it hasn't all been about donations. China has also been able to ride the economic wave of increased exports of medical products and equipment for the fight against COVID-19 (Cheng, 2020). Accordingly, many academics point out that while there may be a component of altruism and generosity in China's behavior, much of it is also bound up with an "attempt to improve her image". (Oliver Stuenkel in Santacecilia, 2020) and, on the other, with the general aim of boosting her presence as a world leader at a time when the U.S. is less present. Likewise, some analysts note that China's cooperation efforts vis-à-vis Latin America are also designed to boost strategic ties with the region in an era in which the pandemic itself forces the countries to rethink how global value chains could be reconfigured, as proposals arise for their regionalization.

Latin America has become one of the new epicenters of the global crisis, and thus, while China's donations are a valuable demonstration of solidarity and effort to forge stronger strategic ties with the region, the scale of the humanitarian and economic catastrophe currently facing Latin America is growing worse by the day, and will certainly require a type of cooperation that will transcend donations of supplies and give countries access to the economic and technical support they need to jumpstart their economies and shore up their health systems.

That said, the question becomes inevitable of , Would China be prepared to go one step further and condone the external debt of the most burdened Latin American countries, or at least renegotiate their repayment?

Would China be open to promoting a type of long-term technical cooperation that would allow Bolivia and other countries of the region to improve their health care systems in terms of capacity, coverage, quality, and resilience?

At a time when the world is in need of international leadership to foster a new form of governance predicated on solidarity and cooperation between countries, an affirmative answer to any of these questions would bring China closer to taking on that main role, and would bring us as a country and region a little closer to the idea of driving change by design, even if we already are in the eye of the storm.

X. The Effects of Neoliberalism on Mexico and its Relationship with China. The case of Covid-19

Eduardo Tzili-Apango[1]

Introduction

The pandemic of the novel coronavirus 2019-also known as Covid-19 or SARS-CoV-2 has convulsed the dynamic of contemporary international relations and national government structures-the very ones that have faced numerous economic, political, and social difficulties originated by the pandemic. From an analytical point of view, Covid-19 has offered an opportunity for reflecting on global dynamics and the status of national structures, above all in order to comprehend how and why opportunities and/or difficulties have arisen upon having to confront a crisis of global proportions. This chapter has adopted two objects of study in respect of the areas impacted by Covid-19. On one hand, and in the first instance, it examines of how Mexico's neoliberal national structure has configured a state of affairs that has hindered the capacity for buffering the pandemic's most harmful effects. In other words, despite the proposals of the Andrés Manuel López Obrador (AMLO)

---

1. Full-time professor-researcher of the Department of Politics and Culture at the Universidad Autónoma Metropolitana. Member of the Eurasia Study Group (GESE).

government against neoliberalism, it has in fact been the reproducer of neoliberal social values. On the other hand, and in the second instance, it studies how Covid-19 has influenced the relationship between China and Mexico.

For the purposes of this chapter, "neoliberalism" is defined as the intellectual and political program which replicates market logic as the unparalleled response for regulating the social order, and instrumentalizes the State apparatus for organizing such sectors as the economy, education, politics, and health, among others. It does so based on the assumption that the market is the optimum am for ascertaining the wishes of individuals and the efficient use of resources, and, in moral terms, as the basis for the individual's "freedom" of choice (Escalante, 2015, pp. 17-23). It is well known that Mexico officially adopted neoliberalism in the 1980s, in synchrony with the global trend of expanding neoliberal thought (Otero, 2004). It should be noted, however, that neoliberalism was introduced to Mexico in the 1940s in close association with the Austrian School, with the aim of creating an alternative project to the economic nationalism that had emerged under the Mexican revolutionary governments (Romero, 2016). Neoliberalism later began to be applied as an economic program—largely based on the recommendations of international organizations—particularly through trade liberalization, entry into the General Agreement on Tariffs and Trade in 1986, and the growth and strengthening of a financial elite based on stock exchange operations (Revueltas, 1986, pp. 68-73). Now then, on June 20, 2020, it was announced that in Mexico there had been over 20,000 deaths from Covid-19, double the number of fatalities since June 1 and making Mexico the second Latin American country to reach this figure after Brazil (BBC News, 2020). While Covid-19 has been put under control in other countries of the world, particularly in China, it seems that the pandemic has had a much deeper impact on Mexico. This situation has enabled China, precisely, to carry out "mask diplomacy" by supplying medical equipment through the China-Mexico "air bridge".

By June 16, 2020, the air bridge had enabled the Mexican government to acquire 1.2 million pairs of examination gloves, 1.5 million KN95 masks, 16.3 million surgical mouth covers, 527,000 protective masks, 416 pairs of goggles, 616 ventilators, 300,000 PCR tests, 40,000 test collection and transport packages, and 9 m3 of melblown microfiber rolls for fabricating KN95 masks (SRE, 2020a). In addition, it allowed the return of 54 Mexican men and women who had been stranded in China due to the commercial flight restrictions. The urgent acquisition of medical equipment by the Mexican government is a direct repercussion of the neoliberal policies applied in Mexico. In 2019, the budget allocation to the health sector was cut by 3.2% with respect to the previous year. This was linked to the federal withholding of 2.5 billion Mexican pesos originally earmarked for various health institutes and hospitals (Sánchez, 2019). The neoliberal policies of the López Obrador administration will be detailed further on, but it should be emphasized that the abandonment of the health sector as a consequence of neoliberalism in Mexico has implied two phenomena, studied in this writing: the intensification of Covid-19's negative impacts on Mexico, and, parallel to this, it has determined new conditions for the strengthening of the China-Mexico relationship. Neoliberalism has influenced the configuration of the health and social sectors in such a way that, on one hand, it has deprived the public health sector, in its character as a public good, of any capacity to successfully cope with a health crisis-such as Covid-19-and, on the other, it has created a false idea of "freedom" in Mexican society. This largely explains the ramping up of the infection rate, as the Mexican government responded with lax, even contradictory measures, to the pandemic, while Mexican society continued daily life as usual, paying scant attention to the recommendations for confinement. In this conjuncture, China exploited the lag in the official response and boosted its relationship with Mexico, a situation that the Mexican government has taken advantage of to serve the AMLO administration's agenda. This chapter is divided into three sections that back the rationale for the above argument. The first section analyzes the impact of neoliberalism on the health sector in Mexico, as well as how Mexican society has responded to

Covid-19. The second section presents an analysis of the China-Mexico relationship, particularly in light of the pandemic. The third section offers a series of final considerations that are the product of this reflection, in addition to formulating research questions that may well serve to deepen this analytical exercise.

Covid-19 and Neoliberalism: A Recipe for Disaster

In Mexico, the health sector is one of the most affected by neoliberal policies. Various authors agree that neoliberal policies in the health sector-implemented since the 1980s-have introduced a market logic that has translated into restricting the role of the State in the provision of health care as a public good, applying the logic of market competition to health workers, reducing public spending on health to deal with economic crises, and the decentralization of health services (Laurell, 2015, p. 254; Krasniak et al., 2019). The effects of the decentralization of health services are deserving of emphasis. According to Homedes & Ugalde (2005, p. 216-217), the decentralization took place in two stages, coinciding in fact with two serious economic recessions (in 1983 and 1994). One of its key characteristics was the decentralization of responsibilities but not of the budget. This exacerbated the unequal access to health services, especially among the most vulnerable population, and although the promotion since 2004 of the so-called "Seguro

Popular"(People's Insurance) aimed to remedy this situation, by 2019, 20% of the general population still had no access to medical services (Krasniak et al., 2019).

This meant that in the first decade of the 21st century in Mexico, there was more private than public health spending. The global financial recession of 2008-2010 exerted a major impact on this trend, since in these years the pace of per capita government spending fell to an average annual growth rate of 4%, while private spending contracted to an average of -2.6% per year. As shown by the study of Calderon & Carbajal (2015), neoliberal policies affected Mexico to such an extent that, at the time of the recession, the ideological fetters of neoliberalism had to be loosened to promote the return of the State via neo-Keynesian policies in order to reactivate the economy. In terms of health, however, the animus of the Mexican state remained particularly neoliberal. From 2011 to 2017, per capita government expenditure fell 0.04% per annum on average, and private spending fell 1.8% in the same period.

Chart No. 1. Percentage growth of per capita health expenditure in Mexico, 2000-2017

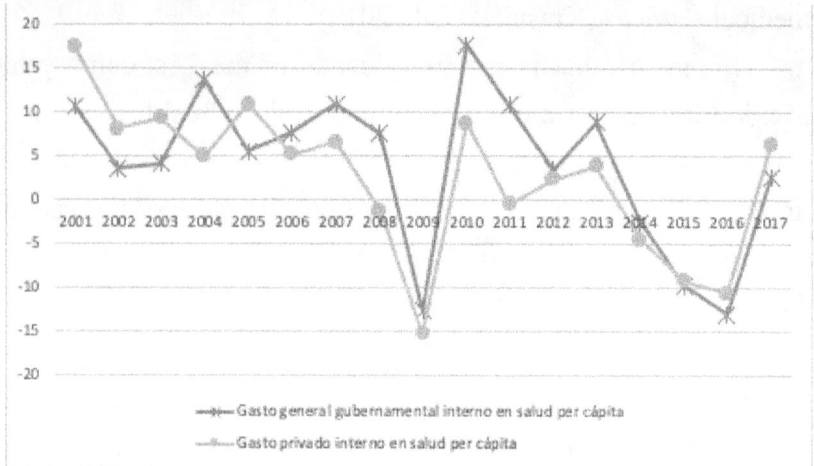

Source: Prepared by the authors based on World Bank data (2019).

Now then, during the López Obrador administration, government involvement in health has decreased; and this aside, the structural problems have continued. It should be noted at the outset that public health expenditure figures remain well below the internationally recommended levels. From 2010 to 2020, on average, 2.7% of Mexico's gross domestic product (GDP) has been allocated to the health sector, although from 2018 to 2020-i.e., in the time elapsed since the start of the Lopez Obrador administration-the allocation has been 2.5% (Mendez, 2019). Against this backdrop, the internationally recommended minimum allocation for universal health coverage is 6% of GDP. By 2020, while the Federal Expenditure Budget increased the budget for the health sector by 2.1% over that of the previous year, most of this increase was concentrated in the social security institutions that provide health care to formal workers, while the budget increase for the uninsured population stands at around 0.42% (CIEP, 2019, p. 30). This contradicts the Obrador government rhetoric that its priority was to serve the population with no social security. This was the scenario that was confronted by the arrival of the novel coronavirus in 2019. As established by Nájera (2020, p. 105), the largest number of confirmed infected in Mexico has been registered precisely in the Ministry of Health system, where people without social security coverage go. To provide the reader with a basis for comparison, as of April 18, 2020 (day 50 since the beginning of the pandemic in Mexican territory), the number of confirmed infections had exceeded 7,000 cases, while in China the peak of just over 80,000 confirmed cases had been reached.

In China, day 50 counting from the start of the pandemic was March 2.[2] For Mexico, day 50 meant the beginning of Phase 3, when the measures of the so-called Jornada Nacional de Sana Distancia (National Healthy Distance Day) were intensified, i.e., refraining from greeting people by hugging and kissing them, suspending public events and classes in schools where there

2. The reasons for a China-Mexico comparison are: (a) it relates directly to the chapter's analysis, and (b) China is the country where the pandemic first emerged. "Day 1" was established based on the date when initial notification was received of 27 Covid-19 cases in China on December 26, 2019.

were active outbreaks, as well as the activities in workplaces where there were likewise active outbreaks (Miranda et al., 2020). However, by day 75 of the pandemic in both countries, Mexico's confirmed infections had increased by 436%, reaching a little over 40,000 cases by May 13, while in China the confirmed infections rose just 2.1%, totaling nearly 82,000 cases by March 27.

Chart No. 2. Comparison of confirmed cases in China and Mexico

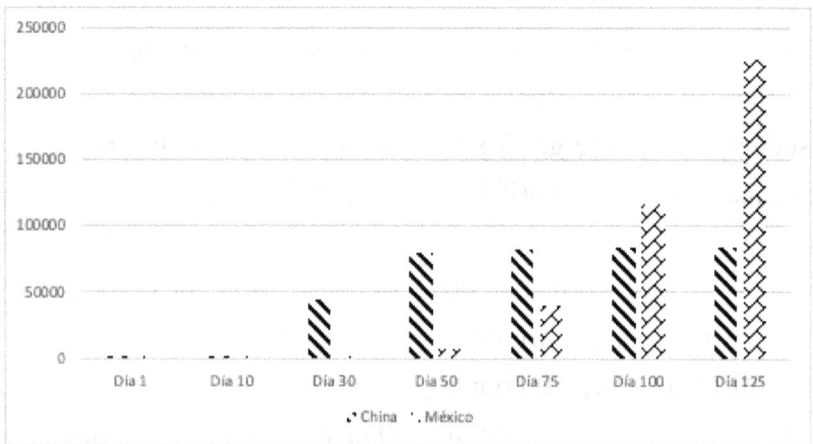

What are the reasons for this gap between China and Mexico? It should be noted that the Asian country's population is ten times that of the Latin American country. Precisely, part of the rationale presented in this chapter revolves around the societal effects in Mexico of neoliberalism, which, together with the global proliferation of post-modernity, has contributed to the disintegration of meta-narratives while assigning preferential status to micro-narratives (Vásquez, 2011), the very ones that affirm as truths only the conceptions of individuals, and no longer those that emerge from within society. Thus it would seem that, among the members of Mexican "society", the proliferation of the ideas of individual freedom and the validity of individual truths has contributed to the lack of consistency in the government guidelines for the response to Covid-19. This may be observed in a party held in Mexico City in the middle of Phase 3 that was attended by 120 people (Excelsior, 2020); the refusal to close down by 23% of companies located in municipalities with high infection rates (STPS, 2020); mass protests by health workers (Expansión Política, 2020); and crowds of people in the fast food stores celebrating Children's Day (Noticieros Televisa, 2020) and Mother's Day (Efe, 2020). In other words, Mexicans apparently preferred to heed their own judgment rather than the government's in relation to Covid-19. Needless to say, on day 75 from the start of the pandemic, with an already historical high of confirmed infections, the Mexican government announced the return to activities based on a "new normal" (Pérez & Meza, 2020). Moreover, López Obrador's neoliberalism was manifested in his criticism of the "Quédate en casa, quédate vivo" (Stay Home, Stay Alive) campaign as "authoritarian", affirming that, "freedom is superior to any other mandate" (Muñoz & Urrutia, 2020). From day 75 to day 100 of the pandemic, confirmed cases in Mexico rose 191%, while at the same stage in China they had increased by merely 2.3%. At the time of writing this chapter (June 27, 2020), day 120 of the pandemic, the confirmed cases in Mexico have risen 93% compared to day 100, while in China the rise was just 0.2%. In sum, neoliberalism has been disastrous for combating Covid-19 in Mexico, not only because of the health system's fragmentation or the "lukewarm" actions of a government that does not wish to fall into "authoritarianism", but because the prevailing neoliberal ideology in Mexican society leads individuals to assign greater weight to their personal judgments than to those of society or the government vis-à-vis the fight against the pandemic, and this translates into non-observance of the recommendation to be quarantined. Throughout this process, one player that seems to be taking advantage of the conjuncture is, precisely, China.

Covid-19 in China-Mexico Relations: An Ingredient for Rapprochement

The López Obrador government inaugurated a new era of unfounded optimism concerning the Sino-Mexican relationship, a perception that stemmed above all from the meeting between AMLO and the former Chinese ambassador to Mexico, Qiu Xiaoqi, after the confirmation of Obrador's electoral victory. At the meeting a dialogue took place regarding strategies for reducing Mexico's trade deficit with China (AMLO, 2018). Within the current scenario of the Sino-U.S. trade war, there have been statements made by important figures such as the current Mexican Ambassador to China, José Luis Bernal, or the Undersecretary of Foreign Trade, Luz María de la Mora, that the Sino-Mexican relationship "has never been better", and that "Mexico can become stronger with China" (Gómez, 2019; Morales, 2019). The rapprochement with China has turned out to be more beneficial for her than for Mexico. The AMLO administration has not entered into the debate on the origin of the pandemic, as has happened, for example, in Washington. At the same time, it has pushed for important economic contracts for Chinese companies, such as the investment in Petróleos Mexicanos (AFP, 2020) or the invitation to tender for the construction of the "Tren Maya" (De la Rosa, 2020), besides agreeing to promote the China "country brand" before government agencies (DDM, 2019; SE, 2020). Conversely, there are no similar agreements for the benefit of Mexico. In this regard, it is important to emphasize that, to date, the AMLO administration has distanced itself from its predecessors vis-à-vis how to manage the bilateral relationship, and in effect, Covid-19 has presupposed a context of political opportunity for China and for Mexico.

The history of Sino-Mexican relations has been marked by discrimination and ignorance, especially on the part of the

Mexican government. Using narratives of periods of pandemics as points of reference, and according to several studies (Cornejo, 2008; 2013, Cornejo, Haro & León-Manríquez, 2013), the Mexican government's response to the outbreaks in China and Mexico of Severe Acute Respiratory Syndrome (SARS) and the Influenza A (H1N1) pandemic-also called the H1N1/09 virus-was quite erratic. The SARS outbreak was seen by Mexico as an opportunity to boost the competitiveness of Mexican products with those of China in third-party markets, although ultimately it failed to exploit the opportunity (Bloomberg, 2003). Furthermore, there was a display of "anti-China racism" with the quarantining Chinese trainers, in spite of their having certificates of good health. Regarding AH1N1, the quarantine of nearly a hundred Mexicans by the Chinese government prompted angry protests from Mexico, even allegations of lack of transparency in Chin's handling of the data when SARS broke out, bringing the bilateral relationship to its lowest point in recent history (Cornejo, 2013). In contrast, Covid-19 has not seen a repeat of historical animosities affecting the bilateral relationship. That is to say, that on the Mexican side no pronouncements have been made regarding the origin of the corona virus; neither has attention been drawn to Chinese nationals, besides which measures have been put in place for bilateral cooperation in medical and health-related matters. On the Chinese side, and in relation to this last point, China has found a partner in Mexico in so-called "mask diplomacy", a foreign policy exercise that, it should be recalled, began in 2009 with Mexico, precisely in reference to the AH1N1 pandemic (Verma, 2020). In the case of Covid-19, the governments of China and Mexico have made much of the "air bridge" set up to transport medical supplies to Mexico from China. According to Granados (2020), it is enabling the Latin American country to remedy certain constraints of the health sector for responding to Covid-19-derived from the impact of neoliberalism-while for China, these actions of diplomacy enable it to rectify the negative global perception of the initial measures implemented by the Chinese government against the pandemic, in addition to helping to construct an identity as a "responsible world power". In sum, Covid-19 seems to be a timely ingredient for strengthening bilateral rapprochement, since it translates into a political opportunity into which to channel the political will of both countries' governments. Nonetheless, it seems that China is making more of this opportunity than Mexico, because the Obrador government's priorities have mainly focused on internal affairs and, secondarily, on its ties with the U.S., particularly because of T-MEC, the new trade treaty with the U.S. and Canada. This was reflected, for example, in the announcement and subsequent recantation by the Ministry of Economy regarding the possibility of establishing a China-Mexico free trade agreement (Figueroa, 2020; Robles, 2020).

Final Considerations

To close the present chapter, some forward-looking scenarios are offered based on the preceding analysis. First of all, given the structural situation as a result of the dialectical process in Mexico of neoliberalism-Covid-19, it is foreseeable that the wave of contagion will continue to grow, and that the difficulties of confronting the pandemic's economic and social sequelae will intensify, above all due to the apparent "gap" between the messages from Mexican officials and the positions they maintain (CNN, 2020). In effect, Lopez-Gatell, Mexic's undersecretary of health, warned that Covid-19 "will not end soon" and called for Mexican society to "act responsibly" (El Financiero, 2020). And while Covid-19 has caused-and will continue to cause-economic and social problems in Mexico, it seems that it has also been a political opportunity for the AMLO government to build an image of a government that "adheres to the scientific method", is non-authoritarian, and respectful of freedom (Camacho, 2020). Secondly, given the structural situation of the China-Mexico relationship, the progress made in bilateral connections could conceivably break down from one day to the next, as has already happened in the past, the most recent example being the Mexico-Queretaro High-Speed Train (León-Manríquez & Tzili-Apango, 2019). One of the most important causes of this "volatility" in the Sino-Mexican relationship is the insufficiency or inadequacy of the institutions that manage the bilateral relations (Dussel, 2018), added to the referenced socio-historical conditions, especially discrimination and the construction of negative perceptions. Weak institutions and socio-historical problems are among the most important elements of the structural situation of the relationship of China and Mexico, which, should they continue as they are, will only yield more tenuous outcomes moving forward. In this sense, "the health silk route" must surpass the circumstantial nature of the current situation and lay down a foundation of enduring cooperation. Thirdly, it is important to emphasize the seemingly contradictory structure between a Mexican government characterized by a low profile in foreign policy[3] and an active international role, upon its assumption in January 2020 as Pro Tempore President (*presidente pro témpore,* PPT) of the organization Community of Latin American and Caribbean States (Comunidad de Estados Latinoamericanos y Caribeños, CELAC), and occupation of a non-permanent seat in the United Nations Security Council for the biennium 2021-2022 in June of the same year; aside from promoting the candidacy of Jesús Seade, Undersecretary of Foreign Affairs for North America, to the office of Director General of the World Trade Organization (Presidencia de la República, 2020).

Within the framework of CELAC, Mexico seems to be

3. See, for example, the first part of the work coordinated by Carrillo et al. (2019).

taking advantage of the PPT to do advocacy for regional actions that could be decisive for combating Covid-19. As Guadarrama and González (2020) effectively point out, part of the work plan presented by Mexico as PPT in October 2019 was the establishing of a priority project to analyze and monitor viruses and bacteria in the Latin American region. On January 25, 2020, a special communique was issued by CELAC on the novel coronavirus, and five days later the First Meeting of CELAC Specialists for Coronavirus Surveillance was convened to update the information on Covid-19. On February 19, the second meeting of specialists was held to share experiences and actions implemented among the Latin American and Caribbean countries. On March 26, Mexico convened the Virtual Ministerial Meeting on Health Affairs for the Supervision and Surveillance of the COVID-19 Pandemic in Latin America and the Caribbean, where, aside from the participation of the CELAC member states, representatives from other states and international organizations were also present, notably the Vice-Chairman of the National Health Commission of China, Zeng Yixin. Apparently, Mexico is strongly promoting a particularly active agenda in CELAC, especially around Covid-19. As for the China-CELAC relationship, however, there does not seem to be any clear line of action. Mexico's plan as the CELAC PPT only contemplates holding the CELAC-China Ministerial Forum in the second semester of 2020, in addition to "following-up on the commitments made during ministerial meetings prior to the Forum, and exploring new areas of cooperation with China" (SRE, 2020b). On the other hand, the People's Republic of China appears to have great expectations following the actions of cooperation arisen based on her "mask diplomacy" in Latin America and the Caribbean, which is added to the fact that 2020 is a special year for China as the 60th anniversary of the establishment of Latin America-China relations (Pueblo en línea, 2020). It is worthy of note that the lack of a clear line of action towards China on the part of CELAC is a structural condition of this regional body (Tzili, 2017), which, unless resolved, could undermine any opportunity for deepening the cooperation between the organization and China. Covid-19 has meant the advent of a change-inducing process for certain international and political structures, some of which are resistant to the change implied by adaptation in order to grapple with the pandemic. As this chapter has attempted to demonstrate, neoliberalism in Mexico has implemented a social and political-ideological structure that, which respect to Covid-19, has affected the society's responses for successfully coping with the pandemic's harmful repercussions; and with respect to the relationship with China, has created conjunctural opportunities for strengthening cooperation mechanisms. However, absent the resolution of underlying structural problems, these conjunctural opportunities will not serve to bring about qualitative improvements, neither of the current state of Mexican society, nor of the current state of the relationship between China and Mexico.

XI. China - South America: Pandemic, Crisis and Scenarios for Recovery

Milton Reyes Herrera[1]

This is a review of the crisis scenarios generated by the Covid-19 pandemic. It takes into account the competitive pressures that are central to the global arena, and focuses the analysis on the reality of the relationship between China and South America, China's prospects insofar as dealing with the crisis is concerned and whether it can assist in the recovery of the region and of Latin America as a whole. Such a recovery should not translate into a contribution to China's economy, and to the international economy as well.

It should be clarified that, geo-economically and geopolitically, this work will refer to Spanish and Portuguese-speaking South America. The region, taken as a unit of analysis in terms of trade, Foreign Direct Investment (FDI) and financing and credit, represents about 90% of the China-Latin America relationship. Aside from this, however, it can also be seen as a unit of analysis because of its characteristics, quite apart from its political and cultural diversity. Complementarily, the idea of strengthening the articulation of South America should be recognized as going hand-in-glove with the possible regional

1. Instituto de Altos Estudios Nacionales, IAEN; Pontifical Catholic University of Ecuador, PUCE.

strengthening of Latin America and the Caribbean, as put forward by Latin American thinker and geopolitician Methol Ferre (1997).

The reader should be advised that this effort, while starting out from an academic perspective, does not focus solely on a revision of the events that have taken place, but rather will suggest possible scenarios, not from a predictive intent (which is not even remotely possible), but from a projective analysis, which is always necessary for outlining viable responses.

Scenarios of World (Dis)order Following the Financial Crisis

In order to comprehend the world order, this approach proposes a dialectical approximation of a historico-structural nature (Cox, 1993), in dialog with perspectives from the Behaviorist-Rationalist and Reflectivist traditions (Qin, 2007; Salomon, 2002), from International Relations (IR) and International Political Economy (IPE), through the approximations of structure of force proposed by Cox (1993). That is, ideas and representations (with contributions from constructivism and the cognitive tradition of the social sciences), material capacities (with contributions from realism), and institutions.

Prior to the pandemic, the contemporary world order already presented a competitive pressure that was expressed superficially and generally in the trade conflict. However it was possible to interpret it instead as masking a more profound sort of competition connected to the possibility of maintaining or disrupting a global hegemony. A historical perspective could also be useful. The leader of the system, under intense competitive pressure that could potentially disrupt the hegemony that assured its firm control over the means of reproducing its power and wealth, promoted the destructuring of the (dis)order that was its own creation. This vision is inferred from the assertions of José Luis Fiori (2004; 2009)

Continuing this line of thought, the trade conflict advanced in the last two years by the U.S. vis-à-vis the Chinese economy will become present in areas tied to competition in technology and the market for 5G,[2] AI development applications; competition in so-called Information and Communication

2. As put forward by Majerowicz (2019), this is imminent. 5G is the fifth generation of wireless communication systems. "By enabling the networked "intelligence" of the productive and urban fabric and the domestic sphere, 5G will provide new, deep and diffuse sources of data production, which will constitute new avenues for control and surveillance (*Ao viabilizar a "inteligentização" em rede do tecido produtivo e urbano e da esfera doméstica, o 5G ensejará novas, profundas e difusas fontes de produção de dados, que constituirão novas avenidas para o controle e a vigilância*)." "The renewal of the global telecommunications infrastructure will make it possible, on the one hand, to deepen and extend the international surveillance systems of the major powers, making room for the redefinition of their borders; on the other hand, this renewal will consume the status of the critical civil infrastructure as a central target in all military calculations and strategies (*A renovação da infraestrutura de telecomunicações global possibilitará, por um lado, o aprofundamento e extensão dos sistemas internacionais de vigilância contemporâneos das grandes potências, abrindo espaço para a redefinição de suas fronteiras; por outro lado, essa renovação consumará o status da infraestrutura crítica civil como um alvo central em todos os cálculos e estratégias militares*)" (Ibíd., 19).

Technologies (ICTs); new patents in science and technology, and uses, development, and innovation relative to big data, etc.

These were all developments that affected the field of material capacities: production—trade—accumulation — investment—finance, security and defense capabilities, and the capacity to materialize the strategic objectives of the countries' political projections. That is to say, the concrete manner of materializing the power-wealth equation. And it is here— especially in the case of 5G—where China possesses a relative advantage, one that from a realistic perspective "opens up an interstice for competition between states and capital, industrial systems, offering development possibilities for surveillance and war" (Majerowicz, 2019).

In this scenario, the preceding reference to North American pressure coincides with Fiori and Nosaki's (2020) assertion that "the world was already under pressure from two major long-term and highly corrosive international forces or trends: that of 'systemic saturation' and 'ethical fragmentation' on a global scale" (*O mundo já estava sob pressão de duas grandes forças ou tendências internacionais de longo prazo, e altamente corrosivas: a da "saturação sistêmica" e a da "fragmentação ética" em escala global*).

At the level of systemic saturation, the space may be pointed out of competition at the global level for keeping a firm hold over the privileged position of wealth-power accumulation *vis-à-vis* associated states, or those perceived as current or future competitors, already identified with respect to their material capabilities. Nevertheless, other spaces should also be considered that allow for hegemony maintaining, expanding and building; i.e., the institutions and their links to the field of ideas, especially to the concrete one referred to collective imaginaries (Cox, 1993), that enable the construction of blocks for maintaining or changing the development model (i.e., images operate in the medium and short term).

It may be pointed out that, from the top position of the system, reconsiderations had been emerging concerning the global regimes and international institutional structures, that were generated as mechanisms of administration of what was termed, at the time, *pax americana*[3] (Cox, 1993). This was expressed, on one hand, as threats and even the materialization by the U.S. of the cut-off or withdrawal of funding from the organization (for example, UNESCO and the withdrawal from the U.N. Human Rights Council in June 2018, and recently from the WHO); and on the other hand, as the argument that China was appropriating the leadership role or the value of the funds being contributed.

Here the following observations are noteworthy:

(a) This is not the first time that the global leader disrupts institutional spaces and agreements that it fomented as a means

3. __Period that may be characterized as beginning__ after World War II and ending with the departure from the gold-backed dollar.

of legitimately wielding its global power, as in the case of the Bretton Woods Accords and the role of the International Monetary Fund (IMF) and the World Bank (WB) as, for example, intermediaries of international negotiations for world monetary and financial stability. However, from the first years of the 1970s and even more in the early 1980s, the U.S. had the capacity to get the Europeans and the Japanese, who were partners-cum-potential-competitors, to align themselves with the flexible dollar system. This finally allowed the U.S. to generate a power of command that was fully functional with the needs of accumulation, financing and change of the production model, while financing its own deficit and trade imbalances (Tavares, 1985; Torres, 2015).

(b) The current post 2007-2008 crisis / pre-pandemic scenario has generated spaces for China's political projection to deepen its ascent and the consolidation of its capabilities for wealth and power accumulation. At the same time it has allowed China to become an interesting global investor and financier, especially vis-à-vis the developing countries, and for the latter to access new financing alternatives beyond the traditional multilateral financing entities.

One can therefore posit that in the pre- and post-pandemic scenarios, despite the aforementioned pressures, the referenced competitive dynamics at the same time translates into possible differentiated deployments of action, a topic that will be addressed later, but that should be taken into account. This, since in spite of the rising strong player (China), the power of command of the flexible dollar system and other accumulated capacities of the global leader (USA) still allow it to maintain a privileged position within the system. Add to this its enormous capacity for reinvention, as in the recovery of its hegemony (Tavares, 1985) after the turbulent 1970s, which had even led several analysts to predict that the U.S. was beginning its decline (e.g., Arrighi, 1999).

General Context of Covid-19 in the U.S. and China

In general terms, we find ourselves before the following scenario after performing a small comparative exercise, taking into account a similar cut-off date; but remembering that here we are evaluating results generated after approximately the same time window of the difficult onset of contagion in each country:

As of April 15 in China (approximately four months after the first reports of the pandemic) reports continued of a total of 3,300 fatalities and an estimated 82,300 infected in all of China (El País, 2020). However, on April 17 China corrected this figure, indicating that there had been an underestimation by approximately 1,300 deaths (El Comercio, 2020a). Thus the total was closer to 4,600 fatalities in the first wave.

A fall in GDP was also reported. It contracted in the first

quarter of 2020 for the first time in China's history, falling 6.8% year-on-year (El País, 2020a), based on information from the National Statistics Office. Growth of just 1.2% was forecast for 2020 or 4.8 points less with respect to the January projections (El País, 2020b).

Despite this, the IMF anticipated a strong economic rebound in 2021 of up to 9.2% (Ibid.), thanks to robust fiscal measures.

As for the U.S., by April 15 (approximately three months after the first reports of the presence of the virus), 23,628 deaths and 582,687 infections were reported (Ibid.), while the IMF announced a possible 5.9% slump in GDP in comparison to the January projection of 2% for 2020 (Ibid).

Likewise, for 2021 the IMF is proyecting growth of 4.7% (Ibid.). However, said growth actually means a recovery, back to similar indicators as of January 2020, notwithstanding the enormous injection of resources by the Trump administration. One example is the rescue plan of US$ 2.2 billion, the largest economic stimulus ever to be launched by a country, which was approved at the end of March[4] (Guimón, 2020). The indicators as far as the impact on the population and on GDP are concerned, seem to confirm the perception of decline; however, this exerts no influence whatsoever on the Trump administration's

4. And that subsequently, on April 24, they were increased when the House of Representatives approved a new Donald Trump public aid package worth USD$484 billion to help hospitals and small and medium-size businesses (Ibid.).

position in regard to the political projection of the U.S. and the acceleration of competitive pressure.

And with respect to China, it is also necessary to note that the crisis was addressed through a number of measures, including the following.

- The role of a strong State that provides financial support to industries and businesses, in addition to, according to reports, new packages of contracts to prevent a new outbreak (for example, personnel posted at the entrance of education centers). This contributes to the maintenance of consumption and demand and keeps up the supply.

- In financial terms China had centralized command over the banking system. Thus, for example, it was announced on March 13 that reserves would be relaxed for the second time this year with the release of around US$ 79 billion. The Central Bank then relaxed the monetary policy for the second time since the outbreak of the virus, to help supplement liquidity, increase the margin to boost credit and promote the economy's recovery. The referential interest rate on loans was also lowered (El Universo, 2020).

- In terms of constructive material capabilities, technological innovation was also deployed, including applications for monitoring and control of possible infection spots and new infected individuals, through the use of 5G, big data and other applied ICTs[5] (which, for example, enable real-time users' safe entry in locations where there are large crowds of people, such as in subways);[6] and supply was guaranteed through highly secure delivery systems, which enabled the recovery, maintenance and boosting at the same time of the economy's capacity related to the e-commerce.

- Control is exercised in the ambit of security, where the State is endowed with robust capacity and traditional legitimacy in everything concerned with maintaining order and risk prevention; in addition, control is exercised by the population itself based on its self-perception as one same community, and as being above individual interests.

- Cultural constructs—Ideas—State civilization that enable "the population and the economy to persevere" from the standpoint of a long-term construct related to discipline, even to values of austerity; in addition, the confidence that originates from the continuum of Confucian character: Individual-Family -Government-State (Reyes, 2018), proper to the founding

5. From the use of the social network Wechat (in Chinese: 微信 , Wēixìn); until the adaptation of facial recognition cameras equipped with software that can scan large numbers of people and spot individuals running a temperature or not wearing masks (Aldana, 2020).

6. The application has the following protocol: "Citizens must fill in some personal data, explain if they have any symptoms or if they have been in an affected place within the last 14 days. Based on this data, the app generates a QR color code according to the level of risk each person runs of getting infected: red, yellow or green" (El Español, 2020).

Confucian principles of the Chinese state-civilization.

Concerning this point, some structural and conjunctural elements present in the region before the start of the pandemic should be examined, and the complex challenges that may emerge in the Post-Pandemic scenario.

South America, General Scenarios and Perspectives: Pre-and Pandemic

Given that the long-term articulation to the world economic order of the region and especially of South America has been based on raw material exports and strategic resources, since the fall in commodity prices that began in 2014, the region has suffered a marked decline in the indices of growth rates of prior years. Likewise, at the structural level we can pinpoint two moments: (a) the weakening of endogenous projects; and (b) the wave of criticism in 2019.

In the former case, since 2015 there has been a change in the correlation of political forces within the respective society-state complexes that has also had an impact on the same correlation at the regional level. We can point out the following primordial facts:

- The revolts in the first semester of 2014 in Venezuela (the exit) that would mark the beginning of a first wave of criticism of the so-called progressive governments of South America; an extremely diverse group of projects characterizable as ranging from attempts at so-called 21st century socialism (Venezuela), reformism (the Brazilian, Argentine or Uruguayan case), popular national projects (the Bolivia of Evo Morales), or neo-developmentalists (the Correa government).

- Macri's electoral victory and taking of office in December 2015 with a clear reorientation towards a project of aperture and a logic of minimization of the State's role.

- In Brazil, Dilma Rousseff's impeachment in May 2016 and the rise of the Temer government, which deepened the redirectioning of the economic policy initiated by the preceding president in favor of an orthodox vision, and disrupted the social orientation of the past administrations of the Workers Party (*Partido de los Trabajadores*). The victory of Jair Bolsonaro and his taking office on January 1, 2019 followed.

- The repositioning of the Ecuadorian government by President Lenin Moreno has oriented it since mid-2017 towards more orthodox visions at the economic level and relations with traditional multilateral credit organizations (such as the IMF, WB, IDB, for example), and reduced the financial relationship with China, consolidated during the government of his predecessor.

In this scenario, the instances of regional integration of an integral type with an endogenous orientation (despite the limitations on the advance of mechanisms at the economic level), with such bodies as the Union of South American Nations (*Unión de Naciones Sudamericanas*, UNASUR), and, tangentially,with the Community of Latin American and Caribbean States (*Comunidad de Estados Latinoaméricanos y Caribeños*, CELAC), appear weakened. The former will suffer a slow death should no new organization be consolidated, such as the proposed Forum for the Progress of South America (PROSUR), while the latter (despite Lopez Obrador's Mexican foreign policy) will not quite succeed in generating the projected that was hoped for in the first years following its foundation.

In this context, the region seemed to reorient itself toward consolidating proposals that could be described as "open neo-regionalism". For example, the Pacific Alliance (Colombia, Peru and Chile for South America, aside from Mexico), with an agenda emphasizing economics and trade.

At the political level, the Lima Group[7] was formed following the Declaration of Lima in August 2017, with an agenda of promoting a change of government in Venezuela to resolve the political crisis. The Group received the support of the OAS, which was then resuming a strong role of processing hemispheric relations, given that in years prior it had lost protagonism in the

7. The declaration was made by: Argentina, Brazil, Canada, Chile, Colombia, Costa Rica, Guatemala, Honduras, Mexico, Panama, Paraguay and Peru, with Bolivia joining later on December 22, 2019. However, only Brazil, Canada, Chile, Colombia and Costa Rica are signatories of an April 2, 2020 declaration. Guatemala, Honduras, Panama, Paraguay, Peru (El Comercio, 2020b).

region, with its secretariat perceived as highly articulated to the perceptions of the U.S.

Here it is noteworthy that, at least in the first two years of this period (2015-2016), a very new scenario has been configured within the relatively new one signified by the relations between China-Latin America, and China - South America. This, given that since 2002 and especially since the beginning of the "progressive" boom, bi-regional and bilateral relations were strengthened, especially in foreign direct investment and the financial-credit level (trade had followed a spectacular upward since preceding years).

This novel scenario meant a resumption of the emphasis on bilateral relations over bi-regional ones (despite documents of a regional nature, such as the second China-Latin America White Paper of 2016, or the China-CELAC forums of January 2015 or 2018), in which China concentrated on processing its interests, taking into account a principle that can be characterized as "to move forward in the relations, and in the ambits according to how the counterpart may put this forward;[8] avoiding-ith traditional diplomatic restraint-any conflict and without proposing suggestions or coercive protection of its interests in the face of the new political projects that the governments in the region have assumed."

8. If the counterpart proposes only the maintenance or increase of trade relations, without a deepening of the FDI or financing relationship, for example, China does not question the national decisions.

The Chinese expansion then continued to unfold at the trade level, new investments were made in Brazil's energy sector in 2016 and 2017, for example (see Annex), and swaps with Argentina,[9] which were commitments acquired since the first Kirchner administration in 2012, were maintained.

At the same time, the proposal was put forth of deepening relationship initiatives that would be adequate for the new scenario, such as entering into partnerships (associations, comprehensive partnerships, etc.); and, finally, the extension of the Belt and Road Initiative (BRI), which has gained the adherence of several countries of the region (regardless of politico-economic orientation, albeit with nuanced positions).

Regarding the BRI in general terms, we would first point out that it already contains five movements that have already been deployed in the region: cooperation, foreign direct investment (FDI), finance and trade, cooperation and political dialog.

Although we may recall that, as a precedent of said extension, by 2017 the Asian Infrastructure Investment Bank (AIIB) "was constituted by 57 countries, including (only) Brazil, Bolivia, Chile, Peru and Venezuela in Latin America"(Zotelle; Wei, 2017, 43), all of them in South America. It was only in January 2018, when China invited LAC to join its initiative,

9. __One amount__ for 70 billion yuans, which expired for the first time in 2012, and in 2014 an additional 3-year agreement for approximately 67 billion yuans (about US$ 11 billion) was agreed (Granados & Ellis, 2015: 44); this was already reached in 2015, when exchange swaps reached a total of US$ 11 billion.

that five Latin American countries, including just one from South America, had signed cooperation agreements under the project (Telesur, 2018). The countries were Panama, Antigua and Barbuda, Trinidad and Tobago, and Guyana, in the Caribbean, and until then only Bolivia in South America. In this resulting scenario, it seemed that this region was not responding proactively to the possibilities that could arise through the BRI.

However, beginning in September, Caracas signed an Agreement of Participation in the Belt and Road Initiative. Chile followed in November of the same year and Ecuador in December 2018, while in Argentina, in a joint declaration by Presidents Macri and Xi Jinping on December 2, "[t]hey emphasized that the Integral Strategic Association between both countries could be extended to the relationship with the Belt and Road Initiative" (Infobae, 2018). All of this informs us of the vigor and speed of South American interest in the Initiative.

On the other hand, the period of demonstrations that were critical of State leadership in the region is noteworthy. They took place in Ecuador, Colombia, and Chile, mostly driven by an orthodox economic perspective. The demonstrations in Chile for the most part began in October 2019.

In Bolivia, they subsequently triggered an unexpected change of government (the preceding one having been led by a president whose project was contrary to the politics of those governing the aforementioned countries).

At this juncture the change can also be pointed out in the correlation of forces in Uruguay (leaning more towards an orthodox perspective) while in Argentina, in December the Peronist leadership resumed its returned to the presidency with a reformist orientation. In Venezuela there was a continuation of Chavism, and in Mexico an attempt led by reformist progressives to retake regional leadership. This generated a scenario where competition from political projects or differentiated models of development was still taking place, both domestically and at the level of the region.

The political scenario was extremely dynamic, while on the economic front, as already mentioned, the pattern of modest growth continued. The economic growth forecast for the region, according to ECLAC in November 2019, was one of modest expansion estimated at 1.4% for 2020 (El Mercurio, 2019). However, in a report dated April 21, 2020, ECLAC recalibrated its data and presented the following projections.

Tabla 1. 2020 South America GDP Estimates

	Crecimiento del PIB 2020
ALC	-5,3%
Sudamérica	-5,2%
Argentina	-6,5%
Bolivia (Estado Plurinacional de)	-3%
Brasil	-5,2%
Chile	-4%
Colombia	-2,6%
Ecuador	-6,5%
Paraguay	-1,5%
Perú	-4%
Uruguay	-4%
Venezuela (República Bolivariana de)	-18%

Source: ECLAC, April 2020, prepared by the authors.

These results must also be qualified by the impact of the activity, dynamism or cooling of the Chinese economy in the sub-region, an important market for China's exports of goods. "This is true for Chile, Brazil, Peru and Uruguay, which send more than 20% of their exports to China (over 30% in Chile's case)" (ECLAC, 2020:15).

However, it should be recalled that South America, as a historical producer of primary goods, could also become affected by the fall in commodity prices, according to the same source (Ibid.). Add to this the drop in exports, especially during the first two months. An example is Ecuador and its important shrimp exports, wherein the following variables intersect: on May 21 it was reported that exports had grown by 54 million pounds between January and April 2020 (recovery in March-April), yielding a total of 483 million pounds, valued at US$1.2 billion, (i.e., 13% more volume and 8% more turnover than in the same period in 2019). However, the sector recorded a loss of around US$162 million[10] (El Universo, 2020b).

In the same vein, given the reduction and re-primarization in preceding decades of the Latin American economy (even before the trade relationship with China acquired momentum, as a result of applying open-matrix perspectives), ECLAC predicted that "the interruption of value chains will impact more on the Brazilian and Mexican economies, which have the largest manufacturing sectors in the region" (Ibid.). The projection for Brazil is 5.2%, and extra sub-regionally, for Mexico, - 6.5%.

This generates a very complicated scenario for the region, in which China can play a proactive and cooperative role for the recovery of the South American sub-region.

Recovery Scenarios from the Perspective of the China - South America Relationship

To address this issue, a few general scenarios should first be pointed out at the international level. At the start of the pandemic there clearly was a consolidation of accelerated competitive pressures for global power that were already being deployed in previous scenarios. Said pressure can also be read as

10. From January to April 2019, exports totaled 429 million pounds valued at US$1.1 billion (Ibid.).

the competition to maintain and expand the hegemony or disrupt it through the interrelations of structures of powerful ideas, constructive and destructive capabilities, and institutions (Cox, 1993), or as competition over issues of cooperation, over how to solve the economic crisis, and over sustaining and expanding the means for the exercise of hard power.

The logic that underpins the above is that, whoever can solve a "big problem" of this magnitude through the deployment of actions and capacity building from the standpoint of soft power (financial, humanitarian and technical cooperation, for example), will consolidate the perception of Prestige and Leadership among the counterparts. In this precise case, a perception is involved that will be understood as the capacity to resolve the challenges posed by the pandemic and the crisis generated by the world economy.[11]

At this juncture, China was already providing assistance to the health systems of several countries in the region, such as Argentina, Venezuela, and Ecuador, and actioning other cooperation initiatives, of which some examples follow.

- Until the end of March, an exchange of China's experiences and knowledge about COVID-19 was held with health officials and specialists from 25 Latin American and Caribbean countries

11. A great Problem that has been resolved through the actions of a power, legitimizes the latter's power and leadership; for example, the U.S. with the Marshall Plan and the construction of the international institutions that administered its power during the Pax Americana.

(Xinhua, 2020a).

- With respect to Ecuador, the cooperation during the first weeks would take place at the local government level, such as the municipality of Quito, that received an offer from Huawei on March 22 consisting of "an auxiliary cloud-based, rapid coronavirus diagnostic system with AI support ... capable of processing 18,000 coronavirus diagnoses in 3 months." (Diario Qué, 2020). However, it should also be noted that at the country level, the Ecuadorian Ministry of Foreign Affairs and the National Health Commission of China held a video conference at which their experts shared knowledge and experiences on the fight against COVID-19 (Xinhua, 202oa). Further additions could be support for the use of 5G technologies to monitor cases and risk situations;[12] and the offer from the Chinese president Xi Jinping to provide "needed assistance and explore cooperation in areas such as research and production of vaccines and medicines to the Ecuadorian president during a telephone conference on June 17" (Xinhua, 2020b).

However, above and beyond the progress that has been made, the following are other potential spaces, directly related to economic recovery, that could be exploited.

- There could be cooperation in the form of preferential financial and credit terms and other related mechanisms, such as loans for oil with optimized conditions, for regional and/or

12. According to confidential sources, per customary practice.

global economic recovery.

- Another possibility would be materializing the value chain and the transfer of industrial sectors to Latin America with enhanced sophistication, as proposed in the 2016 White Paper.

- The use of existing strategic resources that abound in the region (such as rare earths, lithium, etc.) that are useful for developing products related to ICTs, or specifically to 5G, through joint extraction and production, using the logic of joint use and generation of added value and transfer of technology. This would allow the region to recover and at the same time expand as a market, generating opportunities not only for itself but also for China, and expanding mutual trust and long-term partnership.

Regarding the first point, one response from China has been the recent financial cooperation with Ecuador in which, according to the Ministry of Economy, "around US$ 2.4 billion" is expected between June and October.[13] The resources will come from a credit operation and a trade operation. It will include signing a long-term crude oil sales contract to be administered by the public company Petroecuador" (El Comercio 2020c).

The other two initiatives depend on China's political will and capabilities. However, it would seem that, thus far, China hopes to be able to drive the economic recovery as a means to maintain

13. Of this amount, between US$ 300 million and US$ 400 million will be earmarked for the prepayment of the debt from a prior operation with the ICBC, and thus restructure these commitments under better conditions (El Comercio, 2020c).

elements of the globalized market that were instrumental for its rise and consolidation.

With regard to Latin America and South America, it is interesting to recognize that a Reaffirmation of the BRI exists which will have effects on the region in terms of investment, employment-demand, the growth of supply, and so on. To this end, the region should at least propose executing the South American bi-oceanic connection, whose Manta, Manaus, Belem exit could generate, besides the best articulation to the Pacific, to Africa as well, through Punto Seixas in the State of Paraíba, the closest point to West Africa-Senegal; and from there return via Mombasa in Africa to Asia, thus generating a global southern ring (See proposal in Reyes, 2018).

In addition, the possibility of expanding investment and strengthening integration would then arise, as an add-on in parallel to the region's recovery, through the materialization of some of the delayed projects in the Initiative for South American Regional Integration (IIRSA-COSI-PLAN).

Interestingly, thus far China has not ruled out new financial and credit packages for the region. In fact, the Ecuadorian case strengthens the perception that China can partially create incentives for economic recovery. However, first of all she must find mechanisms that allow her to expand her means of payment (since the flexible dollar does not have such restrictions). Here a question arises regarding China's financial potential for a global recovery plan and for the future, of mechanisms that are still being tested, such as the e-Rmb.

However, beyond the aforementioned possibilities and the million-dollar question of whether China will have sufficient funds to lead the global recovery, the developing countries and the countries in our region must also propose their own strategies that will enable us to avoid internalizing a logic of competition in front of the resource scarcity expected in the coming years. Such logic could debilitate the position of the states in future negotiations with the People's Republic of China, and likewise with other global powers.

XII. Colombia: Biopsychosocial Dimensions of the Pandemic: Actors, Moments and Processes

Wilson López-López[1]

In early January 2020, Latin American authorities were experiencing, to a lesser or greater extent, the echoes of powerful social demonstrations in several countries of the region, among them Colombia and Chile, against inequality and lack of services in people's lives. At the same time, China was beginning to experience the impact of a pandemic that would challenge her ability to respond to a major health crisis. Through great human and economic efforts, China succeeded in bringing under control what soon became a pandemic that crossed over to the other continents. Six months later, Latin America had become the center of the crisis in terms of the numbers of infected and deaths. Other chapters of this book provide an account of this. However, in this chapter we particularly wish to analyze the other cost, linked to the impact on the mental health of the population.

In point of fact, the WHO had issued a warning in mid-May 2020 that the coronavirus crisis and its consequences would affect the mental health of many people. The organization

1. Wilson López-López, Grupo Sociedad y culturas de paz, Department of Psychology - Pontificia Universidad Javeriana, E-mail: lopezw@javeriana.edu.co

explained that there could be an increase in suicides and mental disorders and called on governments not to neglect psychological care. The WHO detected an increase in distress of 35% in China, 60% in Iran or 40% in the U.S., three of the countries most affected by the pandemic. La Vanguardia, 2/06/2020. This is an analysis based on the reality of Colombia, though it also examines the events registered in China in terms of mental health costs.

Before the pandemic, the regional economy, while showing improvement in certain variables, had not reduced its inequality indicators, especially in countries such as Brazil, Chile and Colombia, this last with one of the worst Gini ratings in the region and worldwide of 0.5638. According to ECLAC's 2019 Annual Report on the social conditions in the region, 30.1% of its population was living under the poverty line in 2018, and 10.7% was living in extreme poverty in Colombia. According to the figures of the National Department of Statistics (DANE), over 13 million people were living in poverty and around 3.5 million people in extreme poverty. That is, close to 35% of the population was living either in poverty or in extreme poverty (Becerra, 2019). The latest analyses indicate that these figures will worsen as a result of the pandemic, more so considering that so-called informal employment in Colombia exceeds 53%, and all indicators would seem to predict that unless urgent macroeconomic measures are adopted to address these structural flaws in the region's political economy, and especially in that of Colombia, unemployment will soon be exceeding 25%.

It is evident that, at the very least, the countries will have to think about how to reallocate budgets to strengthen health systems, food security, investment in education, and even consider a basic income for the most vulnerable segments of their populations. Independently of whether the countries are led by governments that claim to defend political ideas of the right or the left, there do not seem to be other alternatives to prevent the consequences of the catastrophe we are living through from triggering indicators associated with uncontrollable escalations of violence (Velandia & López-López, 2020).

What is systematically emerging are the biopsychosocial conditions and consequences (DePierro, Lowe, & Katz, 2020; Holmes et al, 2020; Molina, 2020) derived from the pandemic (contagion, coping with the disease, recovery or death), the containment processes associated with quarantines (times and conditions of isolation), venturing outside (environmental, socio-economic, political, cultural and safety conditions, among others), the entering into quarantines, and the "new normal" (after pandemic control, vaccine discovery, and global vaccination).

In all of the above, the weaknesses of our societies have been exposed that have been caused by deep socio-economic inequalities, vulnerabilities occasioned by democracies captured by groups that impose the group's interests on the social majority.

In Colombia, specifically, according to Sanabria et al. (2020) in collaboration with the Colombian Psychological Association (Colegio Colombiano de Psicólogos), from a sampling of over 18,000 persons, the foregoing has been confirmed by the findings in a study entitled "Effects on the mental health of the Colombian population during the COVID-19 pandemic" (*Efectos en la salud mental de la población colombiana durante la pandemia del COVID-19*). In all the regions of the country there is a clear concern for the decline in economic income (65%) and employment (63%). There is a decline in physical activity and sleep habits (50%), 29% of people present anxiety, 35% depression, 31% somatization, and 21% report loneliness. At the same time, a few positive elements are also reported, such as better relationships with others (60%), increased appreciation for life (82%), and resilience (45%).

These data are also consistent with another national study by Fundación Crecer and the company Cifras y Conceptos on a sample of 1,848 persons, that reported other biopsychosocial impacts: high levels of anxiety (over 51%), depression (18%), and "fear of death" (21%). Alcohol consumption is reported in 85% of the population sample; couple relationships have been affected-26% report conflicts and 27% report aggressiveness between partners (Cifras y Conceptos, 2020). At the time of evaluation it seemed evident that the biopsychosocial impacts were indisputable in the two studies and that they are consistent with studies conducted in other countries of the world.

However, the world seems to have forgotten the "before" of the pandemic and the multidimensional economic, political and legal conditions (López-López, 2020)(Figure 1).

Figure 1. The Multidimensional Lattice

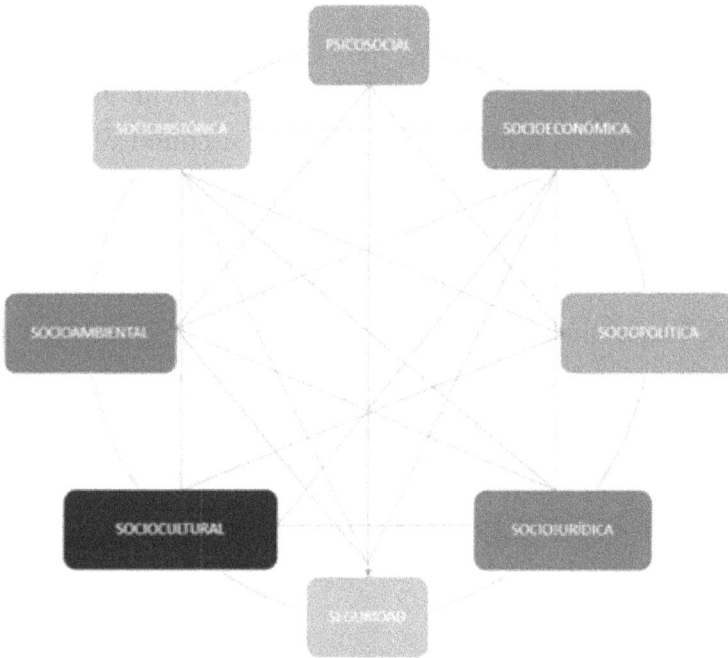

At present, a significant number of Latin American governments have limited and weak health infrastructure, privatized health systems with elitist costs, that emerged when lawmakers yielded to the pressure from international lobbies of pharmaceutical companies and major economic groups that ultimately converted the right to health into a business. Unfortunately, this deepened the inequalities that exacerbated and triggered the crisis. Even less attention has been given to biopsychosocial health, misnamed "mental health", within these systems. We have witnessed the lack of long-term policies for biopsychosocial (mental) health in the states and societies. There is a lack of continuity in the regulations implemented and a marked emphasis on a notion of "mental" health that pathologizes it, in which the medical model waits to intervene only when the worst-case scenario presents itself and one is already faced by the most acute phase of the crisis. Unfortunately there is no perspective of prevention and promotion of biopsychosocial health, and the inclusion of such a perspective is undoubtedly an imperative. Figure 2 shows a representation of this type of perspective in order to help better understand it (López-López 2020).

Figure 2. The Perspective of Biopsychosocial Unity

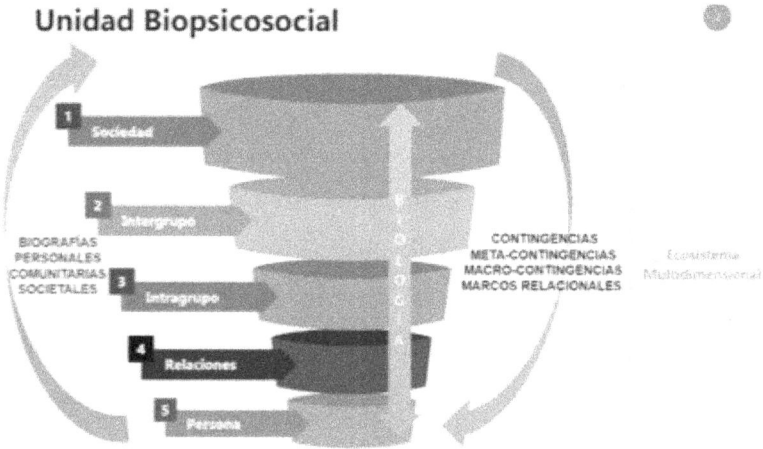

Source: Prepared by the authors.

Against the backdrop of the pandemic, Joshua Morganstein, president of the U.S. Committee of Psychiatric Associations, affirmed that the "costs deriving from mental health consequences will be more devastating than those deriving from consequences of physical health" (Estern, 2020). It should be noted health is still seen in this statement in terms of costs. This scenario is further aggravated by the seeming incapacity of political decision makers to assimilate the seriousness of the crisis. They invest minimal amounts in psychosocial (mental) reconstruction and in general render it invisible or conceive it as collateral damage exerting minimal impact, disregarding the overwhelming evidence in international studies that the problems of depression, anxiety, and all the derivatives of post-traumatic stress generated by this catastrophe will increase exponentially.

Moments and Characteristics of the Catastrophe

Consequently, it is evident that it is from a multidimensional contextualization that we must approach the the comprehension of the crisis, the search for solutions and the development of proposals. The characteristics of this disaster are different and, moreover, have at least five different phases that must be identified (See Figure 3).

Figure 3. Moments of the Pandemic

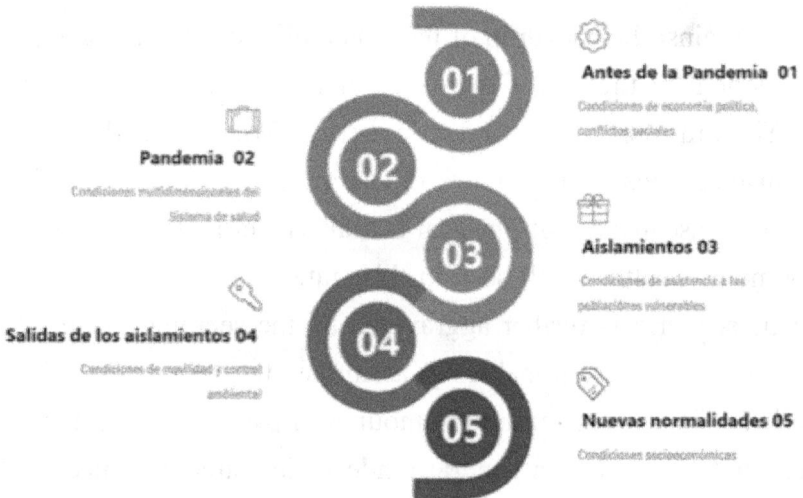

Antes de la Pandemia 01
Condiciones de economía política, conflictos sociales

Pandemia 02
Condiciones multidimensionales del Sistema de salud

Aislamientos 03
Condiciones de asistencia a las poblaciones vulnerables

Salidas de los aislamientos 04
Condiciones de movilidad y control ambiental

Nuevas normalidades 05
Condiciones socioeconómicas

Source: Prepared by the authors.

The first moment, which is pre-pandemic, refers to the multidimensional conditions of the societies prior to the pandemic that are described in Figure 1. The second is associated with the ambit of health, as a result of the contagion, the risk to life caused by it, surviving the epidemic, and the consequences for the family and loved ones of the deaths of those who do not survive. The third moment is related to the confinements, i.e., loss of control over freedom of movement and all its consequences (Purssell, Gould, & Chudleigh, 2020). The fourth involves everything related to going outside, in which conditions arise that are similar to post-traumatic stress. The fifth and last moment is the call for a new normality, in which the consequences of the economic depression are experienced with its sequelae in terms of unemployment, increased poverty, feelings of insecurity and so on.

In all epochs this catastrophe has become increasingly complex, mainly due to the lack of certainty regarding its end and the multiple ramifications of its consequences. This chapter describes the actors, the moments and some of the biopsychosocial processes involved in this juncture, that require a perspective in which the individual is a contingent biography that is woven and unwoven based on the interactions within the relational, intra-group (family, communitarian), inter-group and societal dynamics.

Biopsychosocial Actors, Moments and Processes

Figure 4 is a proposed integrative model of the actors, moments and biopsychosocial processes that are unfolding during the current pandemic.

Figure 4. Biopsychosocial Actors, Moments and Processes

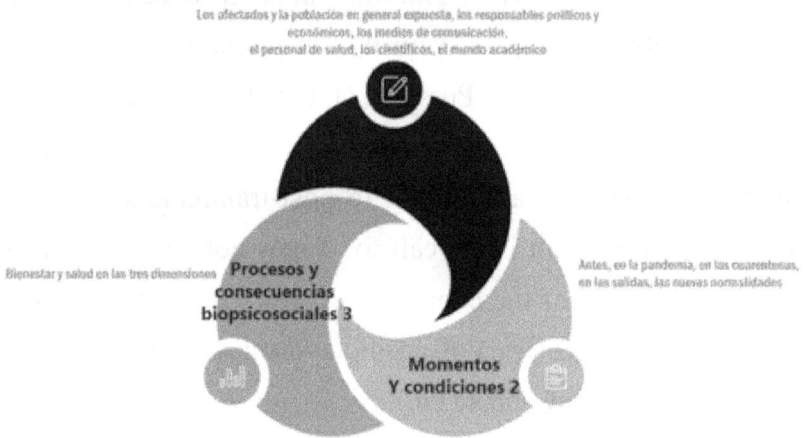

Los afectados y la población en general expuesta, los responsables políticos y económicos, los medios de comunicación, el personal de salud, los científicos, el mundo académico

Bienestar y salud en las tres dimensiones — Procesos y consecuencias biopsicosociales 3

Antes, en la pandemia, en las cuarentenas, en las salidas, las nuevas normalidades

Momentos Y condiciones 2

Source: López-López (2020a).

As the figure shows, those affected by the pandemic, those who experience the contagion asymptomatically, those who are symptomatic, those who have recovered, those who go to the health system without COVID-19, with pre-existing conditions who are at risk, those who arrive due to other causes and do not receive care, the relatives of the various actors, especially the relatives of the deceased, require various types of assessment and, when appropriate, psychosocial care, due to the various effects they suffer that are identified in the studies by Sanabria et al. (2020) and Cifras y Conceptos (2020). Various studies have shown that survivors exhibit different types of post-traumatic stress. It seems clear that the isolation of the sick and the separation from their families affect their biopsychosocial health. And when there is death, it has been shown that the mourning process of the loved ones and survivors is critical, as is the biopsychosocial care given them in the face of loss. It is foreseeable that these processes may worsen due to the impossibility of carrying out the rituals of mourning.

Independently of the cases, the conditions of isolation impact on biopsychosocial health in a traumatic way; the restrictions on movement restriction affect the skeletal, cardiorespiratory and nervous systems; changes in eating habits impact on physical and psychosocial health in general (Addas & Kamel, 2020; Vigo, et al., 2020; Zhang, 2020). The consequences of the latter are more dramatic in countries where there are conditions of poverty, destitution and extreme inequality (López-López & Velandia, 2020), where there is no food safety or access to public services such as potable water, electricity or communications. Similarly, stigmatization of the sick exists as a consequence of psychological and social trauma (Sharma et al., 2020). Society as a whole will be involved at such different levels and in such different ways that ongoing research is needed, so that multiple tools may be generated to contribute to the reparation and development of society.

Finally, there has been growing discussion around the effectiveness of the population's care and self-care. It is evident that we must incorporate the research on behaviors of choice and decision-making behavior of Kaneman and Trevsky, or of Thaler, on how people behave in situations of decision-making, until the work of prosocial behavior (cooperation, solidarity, among others) derived from social psychology (Barreto. López-López & Borja, 2015). This is because the measures of distancing, hand washing, use of face masks, and following society's norms require that society assume a commitment to what López-López (2020b) has called the social construction of self-care. In specific behaviors such as those mentioned, clear, simple, repeated and consistent information is required, and this is why political actors and the media are so important, since contradiction, confusion or the implementation of measures influence the adherence to the norms that are so decisive for halting contagion.

Another group of actors are the decision makers who are generally political actors. As we have seen, at this time their conduct has revealed (more than at any other time) the positive and negative influence that political leaders have over societies' daily lives. Nevertheless, it is good to note how before the pandemic, especially in Latin America, a good number of governments became the objects of massive mobilizations and criticism for their actions and omissions, as in Chile and Colombia, where the citizenry systematically mobilized in unique and unprecedented ways to ask for more equity, less corruption and less violence from the government forces. In countries such as Brazil and El Salvador, governments adopted multiple and controversial measures for managing the pandemic, some of which involved clear violations of human rights, so much so that the United Nations produced a report warning of the threat of human rights violations (López-López, Velandia, & Álzate, 2020; ONU-Mujeres, 2020; Uprimni, 2020).

The rhetoric of the Latin American governments at the beginning of the pandemic revealed narratives along the lines of what they had been doing before, that is, promoting confusing and polarizing messages, promoting fear, hatred and division, emphasizing the construction of tribal identities that divide between groups, extending the in-group-exo group relationship, breaking down social fabrics, building intragroup cohesion centered on the fusion of individual identities around the group, to the point where critical capacity disappears, and even frequently using false information to generate emotions and attachments that isolate communities (Henríquez, Urzúa, & López-López 2020; Aronson 2020; Barreto, 2020; López-López & Velandia, 2020; Sabucedo, Alzate & Hur, 2020; Velandia & López-López, 2020b).

The economic actors are another group of decision makers.

The owners of the financial system, entrepreneurs, are influential and responsible. As shown by Pikety (2019), the ideology behind the models of the builders of inequality influences the political decision-makers who have privatized services. These agents intervene over tax exemptions for their companies, they increase inequality, prioritize the profits of a few over the well-being of the majority, and cause damage to the environment, education and health (Wilkinson & Pickett, 2006). One part of the tragedy we are living through today has affected the poorest communities or those living in conditions of marginalization in a more direct and acute manner. As noted by Garay and Espitia (2020), societies will have to generate economic solutions, at least short-term ones, to assist mainly the most vulnerable population; measures will be necessary such as a basic income for these groups.

In this dynamic of social control, the media, which today manage multiple channels, have acquired critical importance as the entities responsible for the strategies of communication with society. In this sense, we have seen how the media at the service of the power groups communicate in a way that is biased in favor of legitimizing power. On the other hand, states that have independent media have played a decisive role in the dissemination of information. When the Brazil government decided not to provide information on the epidemiological data on infections and deaths, a consortium of newspapers decided to publish the data on the pandemic. It is clear that the media must provide evidence-based information, deliver clear and accurate information to the community on care and self-care behaviors, denounce fake news, and avoid contributing to polarization (Garfin, Silver & Holman, 2020).

Health care personnel (doctors, nurses, psychologists, medical assistants, para-medical staff, etc.) aside from all administrative, cleaning and technical support personnel in health care settings who are in the front line of the emergency, must be protected along with their families and loved ones. The protection must be extended to their contractual conditions, but even more, messages of care and solidarity must be promoted toward society's health care workers. All processes of health and well-being in which they are participants must be studied and rendered visible. There is evidence today of health problems that are linked to the pressures of working in the front lines of the pandemic and possible attacks against the safety of these workers (Gammon et al., 2019). Health personnel are showing high levels of anxiety, depression and fear of violence even in the workplace. This complex aspect is currently under study in various countries. In Spain, among the groups most affected are the professionals who are most exposed to the virus, whether because they work in the health system or carry out other essential related tasks. "Some of them are very fearful of taking the virus home" (La Vanguardia, 2/06/2020).

Scientists are another critical stakeholder group in the pandemic. In the same vein, the dynamics of academic, social and technological appropriation of knowledge and the processes involved have been tested such as: training, communications, research, innovation and development of technologies. This presupposes a joint transformation effort for researchers, teachers, publishers and institutions; ultimately for scientific governance and ethical control systems. The strong developments demanded by the circumstances of the pandemic require funding for research in biomedicine and epidemiology, to mention some of the most important sectors. The changes in processes of communicating this information are also fundamental and should be reflected not just in the speed of publication (O'Brien et al., 2020; Lopez et al., 2020) but also in the pressure exerted on large publishing companies to open up their payment resources and change their model to one of open-access that facilitates the information access of all sectors. Said pressure should be exerted as well on scientists for them to give priority to open-access journals. Similarly, scientific journalists are seeing the importance of their role as never before, in the sense that society demands information that enables informed, evidence-based decision making that offers guarantees for life. Contributions from the fields of psychology and the social sciences have been forthcoming, as has been observed previously, and as seen in the works of López-López and Ochoa (2020), Urzúa, Vera-Villarroel, Caqueo-Urízar, and Polanco-Carrasco (2020) and Salas et al. (2020), and national initiatives like those of Molina (2020) and Moya et al. (2020), or of the Inter-American Society of Psychology and the Iberian-American Federation of Psychology, or as expounded on in Van Bavel et al. (2020) and Holmes et al., (2020) in other regions of the world. Dialogs from an interdisciplinary perspective and inter-professional interventions will be key for the exit processes of this crisis.

Finally, society expects development and reflection from the academic world. The dynamism of the knowledge ecosystems and the developments that prioritize the substantive functions of higher education institutions must adapt in service to this moment, which is not just another juncture in humanity's recent history, but a moment that will last over time and have long-term consequences. In this sense, training (teaching), research and services will have to be part and parcel of our daily lives.

It is clear that previous advances in virtuality in the field of teaching must be fully developed, and the transitions of teaching teams to assume these new normalities must be transformed under the paradigm of remote teaching mediated by information and communication technologies and its implications. The research function, as we saw earlier, depends on the dynamics of knowledge ecosystems, and services will surely have to achieve greater participation in public policies, in debates and in the communications media.

Research in China: References for Latin America

As the pandemic first emerged in China, it was possible from the earliest dates to carry out studies on the mental health of medical personnel, nurses, and other health workers. These workers had to deal with heavy demands, hours of anguish and extreme tensions in the midst of a scenario of contagion and death in the face of a hitherto unknown virus. Psychological support methods were also implemented to reinforce their mental stability in these circumstances. This has been referential for Latin America, where the tensions and psychological impacts of the pandemic only reached their peak months after the same had taken place in China.

One of the studies focused on the mental health status of family members of health care workers in Ningbo, China, during the outbreak of the disease (COVID-19). Based on the assumption that the psychological impact of the COVID-19 epidemic among health worker (HW) relatives in China had not received special attention, it was decided that the study would be a cross-sectional investigation of mental health status and related factors vis-à-vis health workers in five designated hospitals of Ningbo, China. A group of 845 people was recruited for this purpose in February 2020. Information on demographic variables, COVID-19-related events in the participants' lives, COVID-19 knowledge, and family members' (i.e., HWs) work status was collected through self-administered online questionnaires. Assessments of the participants' mental health status were performed based on the Chinese versions of Generalized Anxiety Disorder-7 (GAD-7) and the Patient Health Questionnaire-9 (PHQ-9). Multivariate logistic regression analyses were performed to identify the main factors associated with the subjects' mental health condition.

All 845 participants completed the questionnaires correctly (95.80% response rate). The prevalence of symptoms of anxiety and depression were 33.73% and 29.35%, respectively, with a cut-off score of 5 for GAD-7 and PHQ-9. Risk factors for symptoms of anxiety included more time (hours) spent thinking about COVID-19, and whether relatives (i.e., of HWs) had had direct contact with confirmed or suspected COVID-19 patients. Risk factors for symptoms of depression were (a) more hours spent thinking about COVID-19, (b) more time spent working by the HW each week on average, and if they were parents or other close relatives of the HW. Compared to participants who were health care workers, participants who were private sector workers were more likely to develop symptoms of depression, while government or institutional employees were less likely to suffer from depression symptoms, perhaps because they were in an environment where their psychological needs received more attention. The findings indicated that the psychological responses to COVID-19 have been dramatic among the HW family members during the ramping-up phase of the outbreak. The findings provide solid evidence for examining and attending to the mental health of this population during the COVID-19 epidemic. For this reason, a plan was implemented. COVID-19 specific psychological interventions for medical personnel in China included psychological intervention support teams, psychological counseling, hotline availability, putting in place of systems of hospital shifts, online platforms for medical assistance, incentives, providing adequate breaks and rest periods, a place for rest and sleep, leisure activities such as yoga, meditation and exercise, and motivational sessions [15,16]. Protecting the welfare of health workers through appropriate measures is a crucial tool in the national public health emergency response to counter the disease outbreaks (PSIQUIATRIA BMC, July 2020).

Another work that applies the same perspective is the study entitled, "Mental Health of Young Doctors in China during the New Outbreak of Covid-19 Disease". This was a research study conducted by Shanghai Jiao Tong University and the University of Michigan, with the prior approval of the universities' ethics committees. The research had begun in August 2019 in order to study the anxiety factors in young doctors who were starting their residencies, but halfway through the research Covid-19 emerged, a variable that had not been included in the initial hypotheses.

Trained physicians from 12 Shanghai hospitals who enrolled in August 2019 in the possible Internal Health Study completed surveys two weeks before starting a residency and again at three months (before the COVID-19 outbreak) and at six months (during the COVID-19 outbreak). The surveys were assessed (on a scale of 1-10) for anxiety (generalized anxiety disorder - scale 7), depression (patient health questionnaire -9) and critical workplace situations (4, 5). Mood valence (also rated 1 to 10, with higher scores indicating better mood) was measured daily through a mobile smartphone application.

The study found that physicians in China experienced an increase in mental health symptoms and fear of violence (extreme situations) and a diminishing of mood states after the outbreak of COVID-19. These findings may reflect the additional clinical workload of physicians in training upon the emergence of COVID-19, and are consistent with previous evidence that the additional stressors that physicians face during infectious disease outbreaks place them at greater risk for short- and long-term mental health problems. A limitation of the study was that our sample consisted of first-year physician training in China. Studies of other physician populations are needed to understand the mental health effects of the COVID-19 pandemic on physicians in general.

The majority of new cases are now being detected outside China and it is increasingly critical to ensure that physicians and health care workers receive adequate support and have access to mental health services, so as to ensure their well-being and that of their patients and of the global community. These studies are and will continue to be very important for the Latin American countries (JAMA Netw Open, junio de 2020; 3 (6): e2010705).

By Way of Conclusion

Having a biopsychosocial, ecosystemic approach to health and assured well-being will contribute to more decisive approximations to the new relational dynamics that this situation will impose on us. This is true for our Latin American countries and for other realities, as exemplified by the cited studies conducted in China. This perspective should allow us as a society to put pressure on the various actors and stakeholders to take on board the synergies needed to adequately respond to a complex social situation. By the same token, there must be adequate public policies for facing the challenges that will arrive with mass vaccination and the economic and social crises that the pandemic has given rise to. The academic world will be faced by a myriad of challenges. It is especially worth noting that psychology plays an increasingly significant role in this regard, above all with respect to biopsychosocial health in its many dimensions, the stakeholders and moments that we will live through as we try to construct greater well-being in our societies.

XIII. Trade Interdependencies with China on a New Global Stage: The Case of Uruguay

Ignacio Bartesaghi[1] and Natalia De María[2]

Abstract

The COVID-19 pandemic that emerged in China in late 2019 has given rise to various global consequences.

There is consensus that strong negative repercussions are coming for the economy and trade, with a decline in global growth.

In Latin America, negative growth of -9.2% is forecasted.

The impact of the virus on China led to the cessation of production activity and trade in goods and services, which directly affected supply chains, bringing many industries to a halt. Although by mid-2020 China was showing signs of economic recovery, various countries on all the continents that were directly dependent on trade with China were affected, which led to a rethinking of their trade interactions with the Asian country.

This chapter analyzes the global scenario and the consequences for trade flows with China of the COVID-19

1. Dean, Department of Entrepreneurial Sciences, Universidad Católica del Uruguay.

2. Department of Entrepreneurial Sciences, Universidad Católica del Uruguay.

pandemic, with a special focus on the case of Uruguay.

It also poses the question of how the countries might restructure said economic interaction in the short and medium term.

1. The COVID-19 Pandemic and Its Consequences

Coronaviruses are a family of viruses that can cause disease in both animals and humans, the most recent being COVID-19, the English acronym for Coronavirus Disease. On June 31, 2019, the Municipal Health Commission of Wuhan, China reported a group of cases of pneumonia in the city and subsequently determined that a new coronavirus was involved that spread rapidly to most countries in the world. More than 100 million cases resulted and over 440,000 deaths. There were consequences in various areas and the vulnerabilities of many governments were revealed, mainly of their health systems. The pandemic has generated grave consequences for the world economy. In April 2020, the International Monetary Fund (IMF) projected a global contraction of -3% in 2020. Assuming that the scenario will improve in the second half of the year and the containment measures will gradually be withdrawn, the growth projection for 2021 is 5.8% (IMF, 2020). However, it should be kept in mind that the global growth forecast contains an element of deep uncertainty.

With respect to China's economy, the IMF projects growth of 1.2% for 2020 and 9.2% for 2021, as it is one of the countries least affected in terms of growth.

As for world trade in goods, the World Trade Organization (WTO) estimates that there will be a reduction of between 13% and 32% in 2020, and a recovery is foreseen in 2021 that will mainly depend on the duration of the pandemic and the policies applied by the different countries (Organización Mundial del Comercio, 2020)

The volume of merchandise trade had already slowed down in 2019 by 0.1%, due to trade tensions and the slowdown in economic growth.

In relation to trade in services, the WTO affirmed that it may be the sector most affected by the novel coronavirus because of transport and travel constraints. The International Air Transport Association (IATA) estimated that airlines will be losing US$ 84.3 billion in 2020, with the cancellation of 7.5 million flights between January and July (International Air Transport Association, 2020).

One of the worst impacts of COVID-19 has been the disruption of the global value chain. The high interdependency between its component parts made it extremely vulnerable to the repercussions on the production of intermediate goods after social isolation measures were imposed—first in China, then in Europe and the U.S.—which led to the temporary shutdown of factories and the disruption of production. For example, in the automotive sector over 80% of the supply chain is linked to China (KPMG, 2020), therefore shutdowns affect not just producers located in China, but producers everywhere else in the world. Over 100 suppliers of automotive parts are located in Hubei Province, the site of the first COVID-19 outbreak, which makes it one of China's most important production centers and, therefore, of the entire world as well. The blow suffered by this sector has been due not just to the stoppage and closure of factories and the disruption of supply chains but also to a drastic decline in demand.

On the other hand, world trade was already suffering in 2019 from the consequences of the trade war between the U.S. and China that started in 2018.

It is worth recalling that on February 14, 2020, Phase I of the Economic and Trade Agreement between the U.S. and China entered into force, through which China pledged to acquire US$ 200 billion worth of U.S. goods and services in a period of two years.

The U.S. for its part agreed to halve, down to 7.5%, the tariffs levied on Chinese imports worth US$120 billion. It was a goal that by 2019 already seemed distant, and in the context of the current pandemic has receded even farther from the prospect of materialization.

Enter COVID-19, which has widened the gaps between the

largest and second largest economies of the world.

In late 2019, the first case of coronavirus was confirmed in the U.S., and the tensions resumed.

Among other measures, the U.S. president announced that he was suspending the entry of Chinese citizens into the U.S. because they represented a "risk" to national security.

On the other hand, he asked his administration to end the preferential trade measures for Hong Kong, denouncing the national security law that Beijing had passed for application to this territory. He also ordered the investigation of Chinese companies listed in the U.S. stock exchanges (DW, 2020).

On May 24, China's Foreign Affairs Minister Wang Yi accused the U.S. of leading the relationship between the two countries into "a new cold war," while Chinese Foreign Ministry spokesman Zhao Lijian noted during a press conference that "any statement or action that harms China's interests will meet with a firm counterattack" (DW, 2020).

The U.S. president also lashed out at the WHO for its handling of the health crisis, announcing the end of his country's relationship with the organization.

Already in April he had temporarily suspended financial contributions to the organization, which represented around 15% of its total budget.

This, besides accusing China of having pressured the WHO to "deceive the world" regarding the new virus.

In this respect, he affirmed that "China has absolute control over the WHO, despite the fact that it only pays US$40 million a year, compared to what the U.S. has been paying, approximately US$450 million a year" (BBC, 2020).

Despite the negative impacts on various sectors produced by the novel coronavirus and the aforementioned increase in tensions, there were positive effects felt in certain areas.

E-commerce is a clear example, showing exponential growth through websites, applications, as well as in the social networks.

For instance, the company Amazon has had to hire 100,000 employees in the U.S. to fill orders, while in the field of software applications downloads of food delivery applications have shot up to the top spots (Forbes, 2020).

The same has occurred to Chinese companies that produce masks and medical equipment, especially artificial ventilators.

The environment is another beneficiary of the novel coronavirus, as greenhouse gas emissions have been significantly reduced. China, the country that produces the most emissions, lowered them by 25% in the first two months of the lockdown.

This has been a global phenomenon, the result of the drop in production, the reduction of land and air transport use, and of energy consumption.

The impact on Latin America has been strong and profound, since the international health crisis occurred at a time when the region was already showing significant vulnerabilities and had

had several years of low growth, with the 2014-2019 period recording the lowest growth rates since the 1950s.

The Economic Commission for Latin America and the Caribbean (ECLAC) estimates that the value of exports will decrease by approximately 15%, while prices will fall by 8.8% and the contraction in volume will be around 6%. This is explained by, among other factors, a sharpening of the contraction of world demand (CEPAL, 2020).

ECLAC also explains that the economic crisis in Latin America has manifested in five ways: a fall in international trade, a drop in the prices of primary products, the intensification of risk aversion, and the worsening of global financial conditions, in addition to a diminished demand for tourism services and a drop in remittances.

2. China in World Trade

Since China's entry in 2001 to the WTO, the Asian powerhouse's foreign trade has grown at a rate of 3% year-on-year, over twice the international average.

Exports of goods from China in 2019 accounted for no less than 13.3% of global export sales and 10.9% of imports.

If Hong Kong's flows are added to those of China (which are statistically presented separately due to its special regime), China's share of global sales in the same year then accounts in the same year for 16.2% of exports and 13.9% of global import acquisitions.

This has all led to the challenge of reforms to the global trading system, taking the WTO's experience on board and trying to move beyond it.

Chart No. 1. China's Share of World Trade

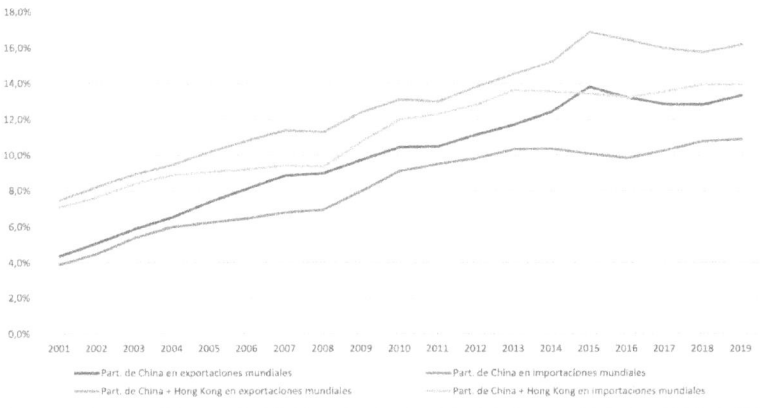

Part. de China en exportaciones mundiales
Part. de China en importaciones mundiales
Part. de China + Hong Kong en exportaciones mundiales
Part. de China + Hong Kong en importaciones mundiales

Source: Prepared by the authors based on Trade Map.

China has succeeded in substantially modifying its productive structure in the last 20 years. This was a process that began with the reforms materialized in the 1980s, in which attracting foreign investment from the U.S., the E.U. and Japan was decisive for China to achieve a new level of sophistication in her exportable offering. China has more recently made a commitment to innovation, with has led to her competing on an equal footing with the U.S., Germany and Japan in the high technology industry (evident in her registrations of new patents, among other indicators).

China's main trading partners are, first, the U.S., as the primary destination of Chinese exports, accounting for nearly 17% of total exports in 2019, down three percentage points from 2001.

Second, export sales from China to Hong Kong account for over 11% of total exports in the same year, 2019.

Some changes can be observed regarding China's main export markets, apart from the aforementioned reduced importance of the U.S., a trend that is expected to continue due to the unfavorable policy in recent years of the world's leading power in relation to China that became known as the trade war (Bartesaghi & Melgar, 2020).

The clearest case of China's changing export relations is Japan. Chinese exports to Japan declined by 11 percentage points in 2019 compared to 2001. Other markets have acquired greater importance as Chinese export destinations as is the case of the neighboring countries in Southeast Asia, particularly Vietnam, Malaysia, Thailand, Indonesia and the Philippines. India's share is growing as well.

With respect to the Latin American countries, noteworthy is the increased participation of Mexico, for whom China is currently an important supplier of intermediate goods and inputs for Mexican industry, which is in turn very focused on sales to the U.S.

Brazil has also expanded its share as a sales destination of Chinese products.

Trade in services is increasingly integrated with trade in goods, and thus it is necessary to incorporate it in the analysis, above and beyond the restrictions still present in the statistics related to this category. China has become an important player in services, especially in relation to imports, since, as the graph below shows, it has a very high trade deficit in this category (close to US$260 billion dollars).

Chart No. 2. China's Share in World Trade (In thousands of dollars)

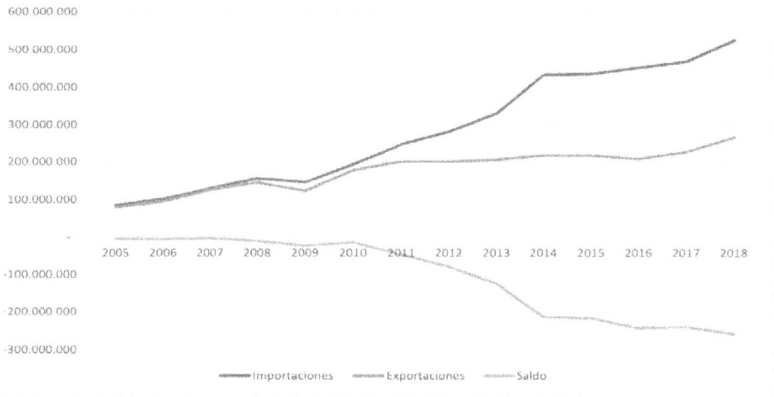

Source: Prepared by the authors based on Trade Map.

With respect to the performance of China's trade in services, it should be noted that between 2005 and 2018 imports increased at an annualized rate of 15% (world imports rose to 6%), while exports grew at an annualized rate of 10%.

The dynamism of China's service imports in recent years is reflected in the space she has gained in terms of overall share of trade in this category, which has steadily risen since 2005 and been especially pronounced since 2009.

At present China accounts for nearly 10% of global imports of services.

Chart No. 3. China's Share of World Trade

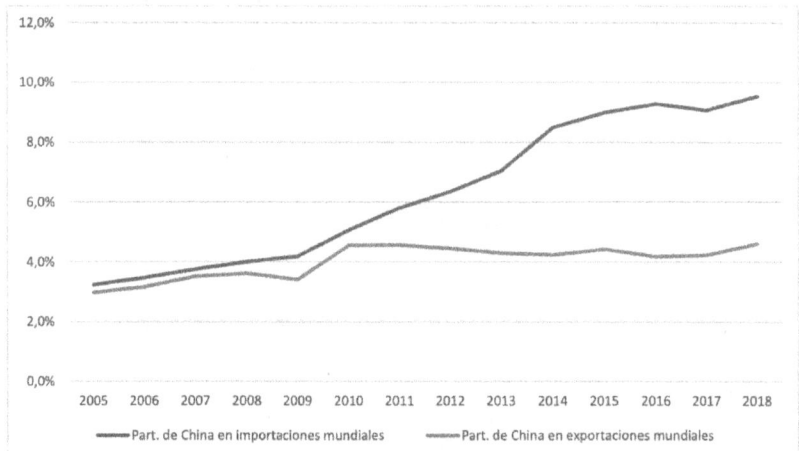

Source: Prepared by the authors based on Trade Map.

3. China's Trade Interdependencies

3.1 China and the global value chains

China's role in world trade has expanded significantly in recent decades, as demonstrated in the preceding section.

The boom in global value chains has led to an increase in interdependence between their participants, but above all on China, as the epicenter of the so-called Asian factory. China has also increased her participation in the global supply networks.

The U.N. Conference on Trade and Development (UNCTAD), estimates that 20% of the global trade in intermediate inputs originates in China, compared to 4% in 2002 (UNCTAD, 2020).

Global value chains had already been undergoing changes in recent times, but the novel coronavirus pandemic has posed new challenges to global production networks.

As a result of the measures put in place by different countries to mitigate the effects of the disease outbreak and prevent its spread through quarantines and other isolation measures, the supply of raw materials, intermediate inputs and end products has been hampered.

Outsourcing, the fragmentation of production and the lengthening of global value chains have generated greater gains derived from specialization, as well as from just-in-time management allowing minimal inventories.

The situation created by the advent of COVID-19 has exposed this system's vulnerabilities, as global supply networks were brought to a standstill by temporary (in some cases permanent) factory shutdowns, along with border closures and stoppage of transportation. Global production was reduced and disrupted, which generated a contraction of demand and supply.

Value chains have been affected from the first moments of the outbreak in Wuhan, an important city for various global supply networks. Besides its importance for the manufacturing sector, today it is a major industrial node that includes high-technology industries (optoelectronics, pharmaceuticals, biological engineering and environmental protection) and modern manufacturing (automotive, steel and iron manufacture) (Deloitte, 2020). Thus, Chinese suppliers are essential for many international companies in various sectors, such that the disruption of production in China generates immediate consequences for world production and supply because of the high commercial dependence on said country.

This strong dependency, besides being made evident by present developments around coronavirus and the commercial war between the U.S. and China, today is already qualified by the Chinese government as a "Cold War". It is evident in the dependence on elements such as rare earth minerals, used in the manufacture of most high-tech equipment, of which China is the most important global producer—70% as of 2018. A similar situation exists in the pharmaceutical industry, as China produces 80% of the pharmaceutical products marketed in the U.S., or is a major supplier of active ingredients.

The uncertainty that is put forth is what the different participants in the global value chains might do in response to the disruption of their production that resulted from the crisis triggered by the COVID-19 pandemic, in order to reduce their commercial dependence on China in the short and medium term.

Some companies that have suffered less of an impact had developed risk management plans for their supply chains and implemented strategies to ensure operational continuity. One way to diversify the risk and, with it, dependence on suppliers in a single country, is to diversify the supply chains or hold at least some inventory should another crisis occur that might create similar effects as those of the present pandemic.

This is one of the most important debates today in terms of public policy, since the current system and degree of dependence (discussed in the following section) make it difficult to take actions in the short and medium-term, apart from the phenomenon of reshoring that the U.S. is advocating, whose outcomes require more time before they can be properly evaluated.

3.2 The commercial relationship with the Latin American countries

China's commercial interactions with the Latin American countries have been observed, and in each country there are differences of scope and certain particularities. Taking as examples the countries of the Pacific Alliance and Mercosur, in all of them there is a clear image of the growing importance of China for both exports and imports between 2001 and 2019.

With the exception of Paraguay, the Latin American countries have China as one of their two main trading partners in 2019. This is also evidenced by the increase of China's share of these countries' total export placements and import acquisitions.

China is the destination of large volumes of the total exports of Brazil (28.1%), Chile (31.3%) and Peru (29.2%).

This is mirrored in these countries' acquisitions of imports of Chinese provenance, shown in Table 2 as ranging from 15% to 20%.

Table 1. China's share of Latin American exports

	Exportaciones			
	Posición 2001	Participación sobre el total	Posición 2019	Participación sobre el total
Argentina	4	4,2%	2	9,7%
Brasil	6	3,3%	1	28,1%
Chile	4	5,7%	1	31,3%
Colombia	40	0,2%	2	9,0%
México	16	0,2%	4	1,5%
Paraguay	18	0,5%	40	0,1%
Perú	3	6,2%	1	29,2%
Uruguay	4	5,0%	1	27,5%

Source: Prepared by the authors based on Trade Map.

Table 2. China's share of Latin American imports

	Importaciones			
	Posición 2001	Participación sobre el total	Posición 2019	Participación sobre el total
Argentina	3	5,2%	2	18,8%
Brasil	9	2,4%	1	19,9%
Chile	4	6,3%	1	22,8%
Colombia	7	3,7%	2	20,6%
México	5	2,4%	2	17,8%
Paraguay	3	11,6%	4	15,8%
Perú	7	4,8%	1	24,2%
Uruguay	6	4,0%	2	15,8%

Source: Prepared by the authors based on Trade Map.

Two differing situations are seen in the trade relationships of Brazil and Mexico with the Asian giant.

Commercial dependence is stronger in the former case than in the latter.

Analyzing Brazil's case, in 2019 its export sales to the

Chinese market accounted from 28.1% of total Brazilian exports and 19.9 % of its total imports.

Table 3 shows the significant increase in China's exports to Brazil and likewise of China's imports from the Latin American country.

With respect to exports, a comparison of 2019 to 2001 shows that export sales of intermediate goods have increased. The situation differs with respect to purchases, with an increase in acquisitions of basic food products such as soy or beef, to the detriment of goods such as those under Item 8708 (tractor and motor vehicle parts and accessories), which were among the five main products that China imported from Brazil in 2001.

Table 3. Main products exported by China to Brazil

Partida del SA	Descripción abreviada	Valor en 2001 Miles de dólares	Participación	Partida del SA	Descripción abreviada	Valor en 2019 Miles de dólares	Participación
'8539	Lámparas y tubos eléctricos de incandescencia o de descarga, incl. los	119.150	9%	'8517	Aparatos eléctricos de telefonía o telegrafía con hilos, incl. los teléfonos de	1.882.794	5%
'2704	Coques y semicoques de hulla, lignito o turba, incl. aglomerados; carbón de	67.675	5%	'8905	Barcos faro, barcos bomba, dragas, pontones grúa y demás barcos.	1.705.752	5%
'2701	Hullas; briquetas, ovoides y combustibles sólidos simil., obtenidos de la hulla.	66.605	5%	'8541	Diodos, transistores y dispositivos de material semiconductor simil.;	1.206.045	3%
'8471	Máquinas automáticas para tratamiento o procesamiento de datos y sus unidades; lectores magnéticos.	52.680	4%	'9013	Dispositivos de cristal líquido, n.c.o.p., láseres y los demás instrumentos y aparatos de óptica.	912.515	3%
'8473	Partes y accesorios identificables como destinados, exclusiva o principalmente.	37.950	3%	'8542	Circuitos integrados y microestructuras electrónicas; sus partes.	758.859	2%
	Subtotal	344.060	25%		Subtotal	6.465.965	18%
	Resto	1.006.865	75%		Resto	29.011.018	82%
	Total	1.350.925	100%		Total	35.476.983	100%

Source: Prepared by the authors based on Trade Map.

Table 4. Main products imported by China from Brazil

Partida del SA	Descripción abreviada	Valor en 2001 Miles de dólares	Participación		Partida del SA	Descripción abreviada	Valor en 2019 Miles de dólares	Participación
'2601	Minerales de hierro y sus concentrados, incl. las piritas de hierro tostadas	744.947	32%		'1201	Habas de soja, incluso quebrantadas	23.075.548	29%
'1201	Habas de soja, incluso quebrantadas.	619.593	26%		'2601	Minerales de hierro y sus concentrados, incl. las piritas de hierro tostadas	22.104.614	28%
'4703	Pasta química, de madera, a la sosa "soda" o al sulfato (exc. pasta para disolver).	143.601	6%		'2709	Aceites crudos de petróleo o de mineral bituminoso	18.520.890	23%
'2401	Tabaco en rama o sin elaborar; desperdicios de tabaco.	120.306	5%		'4703	Pasta química, de madera, a la sosa "soda" o al sulfato (exc. pasta para disolver)	3.580.966	5%
'8708	Partes y accesorios de tractores, vehículos automóviles para transporte de >= 10 personas.	93.313	4%		'0202	Carne de bovinos, congelada	2.094.218	3%
	Subtotal	1.721.760	73%			Subtotal	69.376.236	88%
	Resto	625.473	27%			Resto	9.827.333	12%
	Total	2.347.233	100%			Total	79.203.569	100%

Source: Prepared by the authors based on Trade Map.

There is a different trade relationship between Mexico and China; the latter was the destination of 1.5% of Mexico's exports in 2019, and the origin of 17.8% of Mexico's total imports.

In Mexico's case, one must consider the country's strong dependence on the U.S. as the main destination (76%) of Mexico's exports. Among Mexican main export products are various intermediate goods and electronics.

Regarding Chinese acquisitions from the Mexican market, in addition to minerals there are also intermediate products such as those included in Item 8542; i.e., integrated circuits and electronic microstructures and parts, which have accounted for 17% of Chinese imports from Mexico.

Table 5. Main products exported by China to Mexico

Partida del SA	Descripción abreviada	Valor en 2001 Miles de dólares	Participación	Partida del SA	Descripción abreviada	Valor en 2019 Miles de dólares	Participación
8473	Partes y accesorios identificables como destinados, exclusiva o principalmente.	161.332	9%	8517	Aparatos eléctricos de telefonía o telegrafía con hilos.	3.717.686	8%
8527	Aparatos receptores de radiotelefonía, radiotelegrafía o radiodifusión.	70.056	4%	9013	Dispositivos de cristal líquido, n.c.o.p., láseres y los demás instrumentos y	2.784.032	6%
8471	Máquinas automáticas para tratamiento o procesamiento de datos y sus unidades; lectores magnéticos.	68.595	4%	8471	Máquinas automáticas para tratamiento o procesamiento de datos y sus unidades; lectores magnéticos.	2.196.562	5%
5407	Tejidos de hilados de filamentos sintéticos, incl. los monofilamentos de título >= 67 decitex.	57.668	3%	8708	Partes y accesorios de tractores, vehículos automóviles para transporte de >= 10 personas.	2.093.808	5%
6203	Trajes "ambos o ternos", conjuntos, chaquetas "sacos", pantalones largos,	54.671	3%	8473	Partes y accesorios identificables como destinados, exclusiva o principalmente.	1.721.317	4%
	Subtotal	412.322	23%		Subtotal	12.513.405	27%
	Resto	1.377.895	77%		Resto	33.864.481	73%
	Total	1.790.217	100%		Total	46.377.886	100%

Source: Prepared by the authors based on Trade Map.

Table 6. Main products imported by China from Mexico

Partida del SA	Descripción abreviada	Valor en 2001 Miles de dólares	Participación	Partida del SA	Descripción abreviada	Valor en 2019 Miles de dólares	Participación
8473	Partes y accesorios identificables como destinados.	290.361	39%	8542	Circuitos integrados y microestructuras electrónicas, sus partes.	2.458.911	17%
8542	Circuitos integrados y microestructuras electrónicas.	40.799	5%	2603	Minerales de cobre y sus concentrados.	1.986.013	14%
8540	Lámparas, tubos y válvulas de vacío, de vapor o gas, tubos rectificadores de	33.105	4%	8708	Partes y accesorios de tractores, vehículos automóviles para transporte de	1.027.903	7%
8517	Aparatos eléctricos de telefonía o telegrafía con hilos.	29.504	4%	9018	Instrumentos y aparatos de medicina, cirugía, odontología o veterinaria, incl. los	967.333	7%
8471	Máquinas automáticas para tratamiento o procesamiento de datos y sus	25.416	3%	2616	Minerales de los metales preciosos y sus concentrados.	836.313	6%
	Subtotal	422.185	55%		Subtotal	7.276.473	51%
	Resto	339.091	45%		Resto	7.072.294	49%
	Total	761.276	100%		Total	14.348.767	100%

Source: Prepared by the authors based on Trade Map.

There are differences between the trade relationships that the Latin American countries have with China, but all of them do show an expansion of the Asian giant's export sales, whether of finished or intermediate products.

As the above analysis points out, Mexico is integrated into the global value chains and China supplies intermediate products to Mexican industries that are very much geared toward the U.S.

This relationship has grown so much over time that it was included in the debate during the renegotiation of NAFTA, which as we know culminated with the signing of T-MEC, which set down regulations of origin that add complexity to the incorporation of Chinese inputs.

In Brazil's case, the relationship is no longer solely based on China's provision of intermediate goods for Brazil's manufacturing industry (which at this time is more focused on the domestic market and the region), but also on a significant concentration on China as the export destination of Brazil's agro-industrial products (in April 2020, China purchased 40% of Brazil's total exports).

In recent years China has become a voracious buyer of minerals, fuels, agricultural products and processed foods. Thus, the degree to which all the Latin American countries' trade is concentrated in China implies some additional challenges for the region, since it then depends on China's economic performance.

The pandemic's impact on the Chinese economy has had a strong adverse effect on her imports so far this year. Added to the drop in international commodity prices and the internal crises in all economies worldwide due to the lockdown measures, an economic storm has been generated in the Latin American countries. As a result, a drastic drop in GDP is expected, a rise in poverty, reduced investment and a strong reduction in foreign trade.

4. The Pandemic in Latin America: The case of Uruguay

4.1 Managing the health crisis in Uruguay

Latin America and the Caribbean are currently among the regions most affected by COVID-19, behind the U.S. and Canada, though already presenting more cases than Europe, in spite of the fact that Europe continues to be the region with the highest death toll. The Latin American countries have applied different policies to combat the coronavirus pandemic and have also achieved differing results. Among the varied approaches adopted by the South American countries for managing the crisis, that of Uruguay stands out.

Uruguay has a population of 3.4 million and has attracted the world's notice because of its favorable outcomes during the health crisis. The new Uruguayan government took office on March 1, 2020 and the first four cases of COVID-19 in the country were confirmed on March 13, when President Luis Lacalle Pou had been less than two weeks in office. The new president and his team had to face their first challenge: managing the country's pandemic.

The first step taken on the very day the first cases were detected was the announcement of a voluntary quarantine.

Asked why quarantine would not be mandatory, President Lacalle Pou said: "Whoever seriously proposes imposing widespread social isolation must be prepared to apply the sanctions for the offense of contempt for authority, that is punishable with incarceration. Is anyone, in all seriousness, prepared to send anyone to prison, bring them before a judge, before a prosecutor for going out to earn some money, not for the week (but) for the day?"

The government thus made an appeal to the citizens' sense of responsibility.

Among various measures, primary and secondary schools were immediately closed, followed by other educational institutions, the universities among them.

As the days passed, new cases were confirmed, followed by new measures, among them the suspension of public events, religious services, closing of borders and cancellation of international flights.

The population responded positively to the government measures, abiding by the voluntary quarantine and respecting the measures for hygiene and the use of masks.

On the other hand, the government promoted campaigns in various media to raise public awareness and held daily press conferences explaining the new measures that were being applied and updating the information on the cases. The president convoked an honorary advisory council to assist in decision-making. With over 40 sitting members who are experts in different areas, the council is advising the government as the situation evolves.

Efficient communication coupled with clear presidential leadership achieved a high level of national consensus around the measures that are being implemented. As a result, all citizens and institutions have assumed a commitment to one same goal, which has generated a high rate of public approval (the president has a 64% approval rating according to the polls).

Chart No. 4. Curve of active cases, recoveries and deaths in Uruguay, March 31 - July 5, 2020

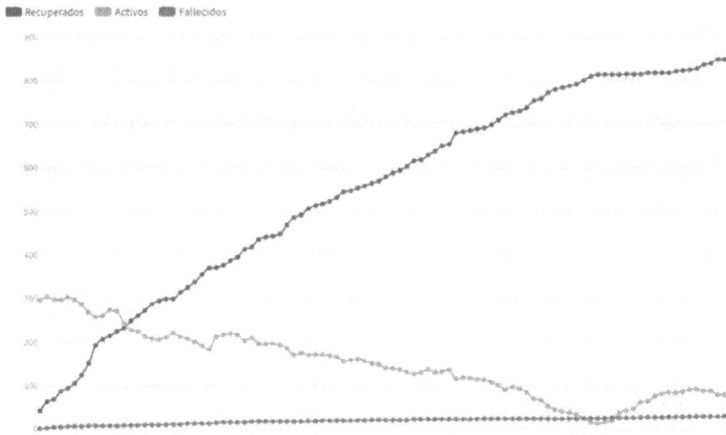

The Uruguayan government has given the situation of its borders special attention given the extension of its border with Brazil, the pandemic's epicenter in Latin America.

The border between Uruguay and Brazil is permeable and

the fluctuating flow of people living and working on either side of it has generated points of contagion, mainly in the departments of Artigas, Rivera and Treinta y Tres.

However, in the capital city of Montevideo, which was the center of infection when the coronavirus reached Uruguay, the situation was brought under control. Considering that half of the population resides in the capital, the infection rate is very low.

Regarding economic measures, a US$12 million Coronavirus Fund (*Fondo Coronavirus*) was created. To help finance it, discounts were applied to approximately 15,000 public officials' and political leaders' salaries that exceeded 80,000 Uruguayan pesos after taxes—equivalent to US$ 1,800—varying between 5%, 10% and 15%, to contribute to the fight against the health crisis. Funds were also requested from international organizations such as the IDB, CAF, the World Bank; and funds from FOCEM of Mercosur were used to palliate the effects of the crisis on employment, the economy, and to boost the social and health system.

Given its good results, the country slowly began to be reactivated. The construction sector was the first to do so as early as April.

Public offices were opened up, trade was reactivated and schools began to open, observing all necessary precautions and measures of social distancing. Another sign of good management of the crisis and its favorable outcomes was that when the

European Union reopened its borders to 15 countries, one of these was Uruguay, making it the only Latin American country whose nationals may enter the European bloc countries.

4.2 Uruguay's trade relationship with China in times of COVID-19

The trade relationship between Uruguay and China has grown significantly in the recent decade and the Asian country has become an important commercial partner for Uruguay. In the first semester of 2020, already in the times of COVID-19, China positioned herself as the primary destination of Uruguayan exports and as the second point of origin of Uruguay's imports, after Brazil.

Export sales from Uruguay to China decreased 42.4% in the first semester of 2020 compared to the same period in the previous year, while imports from China decreased 15.7%.

Chart No. 5. Uruguay exports to China (Not including Free Trade Zones)

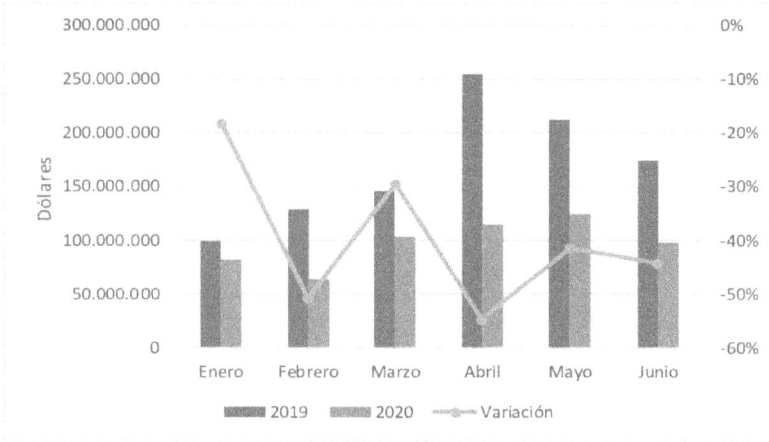

Source: Prepared by the authors based on Smart Data.

Chart No. 6. Imports into Uruguay from China

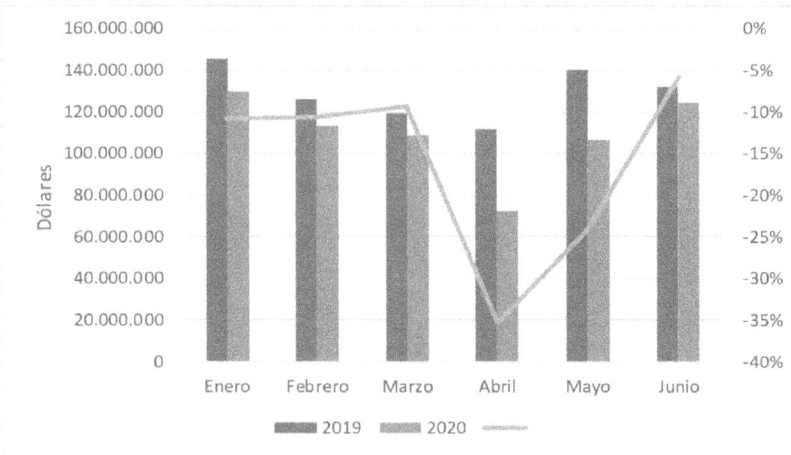

Source: Prepared by the authors based on Smart Data.

If we examine this in product terms, the decrease in exports from Uruguay to China in the first semester of 2020 is mainly explained by the drop in sales of meat (-31.7%), seeds and oleaginous fruits (-71,3%), wood (-40,1%), wool (-72,6%). Noteworthy is the significant concentration of exports to China, considering that the four main products constitute 93.4% of Uruguay's export sales to the Chinese market between January and June 2020.

With respect to imports, observing the main products acquired there is a notable decrease in purchases in Chapter 85 (-23.3%), 84 (-3.3%), 61 (-22,95), 62 (-33.25) and 39 (-44.8%).

Table 7. Main products exported by Uruguay to China (Jan.– Jun., excluding Free Trade Zones)

Exportaciones de Uruguay a China (enero - junio)					
Capítulo del S.A.	Valor en Dólares		Participación		Variación 2020/2019
	2019	2020	2019	2020	
02-CARNE Y DESPOJOS COMESTIBLES.	563.574.985	384.823.826	55,4%	65,7%	-31,7%
12-SEMILLAS Y FRUTOS OLEAGINOSOS.	234.144.263	67.277.909	23,0%	11,5%	-71,3%
44-MADERA.	89.552.312	53.645.119	8,8%	9,2%	-40,1%
04-LECHE Y PRODUCTOS LÁCTEOS.	16.891.088	20.811.029	1,7%	3,6%	23,2%
51-LANA Y PELO FINO U ORDINARIO.	72.833.137	19.949.180	7,2%	3,4%	-72,6%
01-ANIMALES VIVOS.	143.370	10.589.040	0,0%	1,8%	7285,8%
41-PIELES (EXCEPTO LA PELETERIA).	17.667.998	7.519.352	1,7%	1,3%	-57,4%
03-PESCADOS Y CRUSTÁCEOS.	4.825.961	5.974.078	0,5%	1,0%	23,8%
23-RESIDUOS Y DESPERDICIOS DE LAS INDUSTRIAS ALIMENTARIAS.	6.366.650	5.097.131	0,6%	0,9%	-19,9%
71-PERLAS NATURALES (FINAS)* O CULTIVADAS.	3.822.056	2.208.037	0,4%	0,4%	-42,2%
Subtotal	1.009.821.819	577.894.702	99,3%	98,7%	-42,8%
Resto	6.621.533	7.476.548	0,7%	1,3%	12,9%
Total	1.016.443.353	585.371.250	100%	100%	-42,4%

Source: Prepared by the authors based on Smart Data.

Table 8. Main products imported by Uruguay from China (Jan. – Jun.)

Capítulo del S.A.	Valor en Dólares		Participación		Variación 2020/2019
Importaciones de Uruguay procedentes de China (enero - junio)					
	2019	2020	2019	2020	
85-MÁQUINAS, APARATOS Y MATERIAL ELÉCTRICO.	189.138.156	145.108.688	24,3%	22,1%	-23,3%
84-REACTORES NUCLEARES, CALDERAS.	115.556.848	111.717.978	14,9%	17,0%	-3,3%
87-VEHÍCULOS AUTOMÓVILES.	36.498.616	44.132.932	4,7%	6,7%	20,9%
61-PRENDAS Y COMPLEMENTOS (ACCESORIOS), DE VESTIR, DE PUNTO.	42.063.168	32.448.804	5,4%	5,0%	-22,9%
29-PRODUCTOS QUÍMICOS ORGÁNICOS.	33.491.732	30.719.888	4,3%	4,7%	-8,3%
94-MUEBLES.	28.491.940	28.122.430	3,7%	4,3%	-1,3%
38-PRODUCTOS DIVERSOS DE LAS INDUSTRIAS QUÍMICAS	32.408.504	27.261.891	4,2%	4,2%	-15,9%
62-PRENDAS Y COMPLEMENTOS (ACCESORIOS), DE VESTIR, EXCEPTO LOS DE PUNTO.	38.207.620	25.532.436	4,9%	3,9%	-33,2%
39-PLÁSTICO Y SUS MANUFACTURAS.	45.190.100	24.956.528	5,8%	3,8%	-44,8%
73-MANUFACTURAS DE FUNDICION, HIERRO O ACERO.	22.047.077	18.877.433	2,8%	2,9%	-14,4%
Sub total	583.093.762	488.879.009	75,0%	74,6%	-16,2%
Resto	193.908.858	166.420.453	25,0%	25,4%	-14,2%
Total	777.002.620	655.299.462	100%	100%	-15,7%

Source: Prepared by the authors based on Smart Data.

The commercial relationship between Uruguay and China is complementary in character, with the South American country exporting mainly commodities and importing more industrialized goods.

A strong concentration is also observed in both export and import products.

Likewise, the international health crisis strongly affects the commercial relationship, the exchange of goods, and without a doubt directly impacts on the Uruguayan economy because of China's importance as the market for Uruguay's exports.

However, above and beyond the decrease in trade volume, Uruguay and China showed mutual solidarity through donations of medical material to fight the coronavirus.

Not only did the two governments maintain contact and make donations, but the two nations' corporations as well (Embajada de China en Uruguay, 2020).

The Jack Ma and Alibaba Foundations donated 100,000 disposable medical masks, 20,000 diagnostic kits and 5 ventilators to Uruguay to collaborate in prevention and the fight against the COVID-19 pandemic.

Another example is the Chinese company Chery, which made a donation to Uruguay of 10,000 disposable medical masks to collaborate in the prevention and fight against the novel coronavirus pandemic.

Unlike other countries, Uruguay did not echo the criticisms of the U.S. against China regarding her responsibility for the arising of the virus or its link to the WHO, in a sign of support for a strategic partner of the country's foreign policy.

5. Conclusions

The effects of COVID-19 will be very strongly felt by the global economy.

Aside from the significant drop in world GDP, trade and investment in 2020, which will exert impact at the social level (increased poverty), the pandemic has accelerated certain debates that were already underway.

A recurrent issue in academic debates, but also at the

public policy level was the so-called dependency in the trade relationship with China.

In Latin America, these same debates center on China's role in the so-called re-primarization of exports, a debate often encumbered by conceptual errors such as the low technological level attributed to agricultural products and the service component.

Within the framework of COVID-19 another debate emerges that is associated to the supply chains of goods and services, especially because of the industrial blackout decreed in Wuhan in January and February 2020, that was a cause of great difficulties for some sectors of global industry.

The situation led to an in-depth debate on the level of dependencies that have been generated vis-à-vis the leading world exporter, not just in intermediate goods, generating a standstill in the technology industry, but also in goods in very high demand at this time, such as medical products and supplies, a sector wherein China also has a preponderant role.

While the trade in intermediate goods is trending downward in many categories, and on top of this, a push is underway for reshoring through the public policies of certain powers such as the U.S., thanks to technological changes it is possible, and the statistics indicate this, that the trade links forged with China over the past 20 years will be sustained.

Doing so will imply assuming positions that could affect the competitiveness of finished goods and impact on the consumer.

While it does lie within the realm of possibility for certain countries to exert efforts to diversify their trade dependencies, always a welcome prospect, the exercise will be far from easy and China will continue to play a role, not just in the Global Value Chains, but as a supplier of final products that will incorporate increasingly more high tech components, and as a buyer of agricultural and mineral products.

In Uruguay's case, the trade relationship has expanded in recent years and the reduction in bilateral trade provoked by COVID-19 has had a direct impact on Uruguay's export sales. Nevertheless, the relationship between Uruguay and China transcends commerce, and this was expressed through their mutual support in confronting the health crisis.

EPILOGUE:
Science and Technology: A Growing Conversation between China and Latin America

José Luis Valenzuela[1]

In various presentations at conferences with our Chinese colleagues, I have had to raise the issue of the Latin American deficit when it comes to science and technology. Despite certain differences, the fact is that countries in this region of the world have very low statistics when it comes to the percentage of GDP that they dedicate to scientific research and technological advances. And in the same manner, expressions of collective work in the region in these areas are far and few. This was the scenario where the COVID-19 pandemic found us, and it demonstrated—along with other social realities that became evident—how necessary it is to rescue the concepts of "integration" and "regional cooperation" if we seek considerable advances in the future as a region.

We have not planned ahead. And, in a certain way, the concepts of "planning" or "public policy" committed to prospective analysis appear cornered by the premises that, in one way or another, were imposed on the region, favoring market-oriented laws as a channel, where the social issues would

1. Associate researcher, CELC, UNAB

spontaneously find their way. And what do we see in front of us when we look at the reality of China? A significant assessment of knowing where one is going or wants to go: the example is in the XIV Five-Year Plan for the 2021/2025 period. Born in 1953, four years after the founding of the People's Republic, the thirteen five-year plans implemented to date have contributed decisively to the transformation of China, which has gone from being a substantially agrarian economy in search of food self-sufficiency to becoming the main workshop of the world with accelerated changes that make it a decisive global technological power.

In the various previous meetings for Plan XIV and in the consultations before reaching the final proposal, the weight of the pandemic in the current circumstances and its future consequences was present. But here, as in previous five-year plans, China's economic planning was essentially indicative. In other words, the definitions of certain objectives towards which the State and the political leadership indicate that progress must be made are enunciated, but the economic and social actors must apply their own merits and capacities to act within that framework.

Speaking before the APEC Forum (of which Chile, Mexico and Peru are members), President Xi Jinping delivered a highly transparent speech on the paths that China has decided to take for the comprehensive construction of a modern socialist country. He recalled that the Asia-Pacific region, despite two financial crises, has lifted more than one billion of its population out of poverty and has become the region with the strongest and most dynamic economic growth in the world.

But at the same time, he laid down the pending challenges frankly, in which progress cannot be considered positive only by growth statistics but must earn its legitimacy through a better quality of life of the peoples. That is why, from Latin America, we know what he is talking about when he says that there are "growing contradictions between equity and efficiency, growth and distribution, technology and employment, as well as the wide gap between the rich and the poor." In this framework, he raised four points that determine a new cooperation strategy, to which Latin Americans should pay special attention:

a) progress in maintaining open trade should bring social inclusion;

b) growth must be innovative, which calls for training new generations to assume and generate innovation for the benefit of all people;

c) connectivity is essential both for cooperation and exchanges aimed at creating unprecedented coexistence in the 21st century;

d) understand—as the COVID 19 Pandemic and the challenges of climate change show—that cooperation with shared gains is the path of the future.

The Analyses of the II Science and Technology Forum

The Spanish edition of this book went into circulation before the II CELAC-China Science Forum took place, which, along with the various approaches on cooperation in this field, paid special attention to the COVID-19 situation in the region. Mexico chaired, in its condition of Pro Tempore Presidency (PTP) of the Community of Latin American and Caribbean States (CELAC), together with China, the II Forum on Science, Technology and Innovation between China and this regional coordination entity. The meeting, held virtually, was led by the Mexican Foreign Minister, Marcelo Ebrard Casaubon, and the Minister of Science and Technology of the People's Republic of China, Wang Zhigang, to address issues related to development and cooperation against Covid-19, according to a statement from the Ministry of Foreign Affairs of the Aztec country.

Cooperation for innovation in science and technology has played an important role in the development of relations between CELAC and China, Mexican Foreign Minister Marcelo Ebrard said at the video conference. Therefore, topics of the forum's analysis also included "the development and potential for cooperation in science and technology, in particular 5G technology, artificial intelligence, and electronic commerce in the context of the pandemic; trends in the development of science and technology in the post-pandemic era", according to a statement from the Mexican Foreign Ministry.

The summit also addressed what it called a "new perspective of cooperation in scientific and technological innovation between China and the countries of Latin America and the Caribbean, including space cooperation". The agreements of the meeting were set into a Joint Declaration in which "they expressed their interest in deepening cooperation for development in science, technology and innovation (STI)". All this will be done, according to the Mexican Foreign Ministry, "with a social dimension and care for the environment", for which the relevant role of science and technology in the fight against the pandemic caused by Covid-19 is recognized. As this book shows, Latin Americans acted in an uncoordinated way in the face of the pandemic: each one seeking on their own how to stock up on equipment and medical support, while China tried to transfer its experience through collective dialogue with the entire region as a whole.

Minister Wang Zhigang highlighted the importance of strengthening cooperation in the following aspects:

• Development and cooperation of biomedical research on COVID-19.

• Coordination of cooperation strategies, deepening collaboration and exchange through, for example, the creation of joint laboratories on topics of common interest.

• Establishing a common platform to deepen S&T dialogue

and cooperation between the parties.

• Creating a better ecosystem to harness the results of scientific achievements and the use of new technologies for social development.

In the joint statement, the parties recognized the beneficial results obtained through various actions carried out between China and the CELAC member countries, highlighted the respective comparative advantages, and pledged to multiply efforts and intensify collaboration to promote socio-economic development through innovation. They in turn highlighted the important role of science and technology in the fight against the COVID-19 pandemic, and expressed their willingness to strengthen scientific exchanges and collaboration of relevant sectors in the fields of vaccines, drugs, tests and diagnostics, among other common interests. At the same time, they agreed on the following aspects:

• Promote the exchange of researchers and innovators, as well as the exchange of academic mobility, continue the exchange program for young scientists, organize training courses in applicable advanced technology and S&T management, in order to promote the regional development of S&T with a social dimension and environmental care.

• Collaborate in joint laboratories to strengthen research and technological innovation in prioritized areas of common interest.

• Explore the collaboration of science parks, fostering the exchange of experiences and information, to build a cooperative innovation network making the most out of existing science parks.

• Support advanced technology transfer activities and promote cooperation between research institutes, universities and companies, as well as matters related to this process such as intellectual property.

In regard to overcoming the pandemic, the participants "expressed their willingness to strengthen scientific exchanges and collaboration regarding vaccines, drugs, tests and diagnoses", from the CELAC Forum. The purpose of the forum is to promote cooperation in science, technology and innovation for the mutual benefit of CELAC and China, particularly in the context of combating the Covid-19 pandemic.

The final text states that all parties pledge to multiply their efforts to promote and intensify pragmatic collaboration to promote socio-economic development with innovation as the engine. "All parties recognized the important role of science and technology in the fight against the Covid-19 pandemic, and expressed their willingness to strengthen scientific exchanges and collaboration of relevant sectors in the fields of vaccines, drugs, tests and diagnoses, among other common interests," says the statement.

The first Science, Technology and Innovation Forum within the framework of the CELAC-China dialogue took place in September 2015 in Quito, Ecuador. From that event, where representatives of 25 large Chinese companies in the sector were present, to now, the evolution in this field has been of great dimensions. Not only because of the advances, especially in 5G and its applications, but also because of the interwinding of science and technological innovation with strategic political debates in various countries, especially those regarding high development. Latin America feels the urgency of moving forward to a greater integration and a sense of common task in the face of this pandemic and those to come. Scientific and technological cooperation—above political differences—is an area where visions may converge, where the protection of life and safeguarding of the human being are at the center of a well-understood planning.

The Minister of Science, Technology and Innovation of Argentina, Roberto Salvarezza, emphatically pointed this out in that meeting when he highlighted that the pandemic has demonstrated the need to work in solidarity. And at the end of his speech, he stressed that "this Forum has become a fundamental tool, an opportunity to complement and enhance our capacity not only in the area of biomedicine. Argentina has an active scientific community with close ties to the entire Latin American community and also with scientists from the

People's Republic of China. With the latter we share not only the COVID-19 agenda, but also an active cooperation in the area of food technology, space research and in the area of social sciences, which we wish to deepen and share with all CELAC countries". The pages of this book, written from various capitals of Latin America, reinforce the importance of choosing that path: the upcoming world is one of global issues, where multilateral actions will be the only way to face an agenda of accelerated change and challenges which are yet to be fully identified.

Finally, it's worth mentioning how the pandemic affects the most deprived sectors around the world, causing very strong setbacks in the area of extreme poverty. And it is here where it's important to compare the policies applied in China in relation to the rest of the world and especially to our region.

As indicated in mid-June by the Economic Commission for Latin America and the Caribbean (ECLAC) and the Food and Agriculture Organization of the United Nations (FAO), the crisis caused by the COVID-19 pandemic in Latin America and the Caribbean for 2020 could push 83.4 million people to fall under the category of extreme poverty, which would imply a significant rise in hunger levels, due to the difficulty in access to food that these people will face.

In China, despite the leaving behind of the previously planned growth goal, the goal of eliminating extreme poverty by 2020 was kept and all efforts were concentrated on job

creation and social protection. The following graph shows the
global trajectory of extreme poverty as of 2015 in the world.
At the beginning of 2019, it was considered that the goal of
extreme poverty in the world for 2021 could be around 7.5%.
But the pandemic totally altered that estimate. World Bank data
project that the world in a pandemic will have between 110
and 146 million additional people under extreme poverty by
2021 compared to the world without a pandemic. In the best
case scenario, extreme poverty will reach 9% and the most
pessimistic estimate (dotted in the graph) suggests 9.5%.

Change in extreme poverty before and after Covid-19

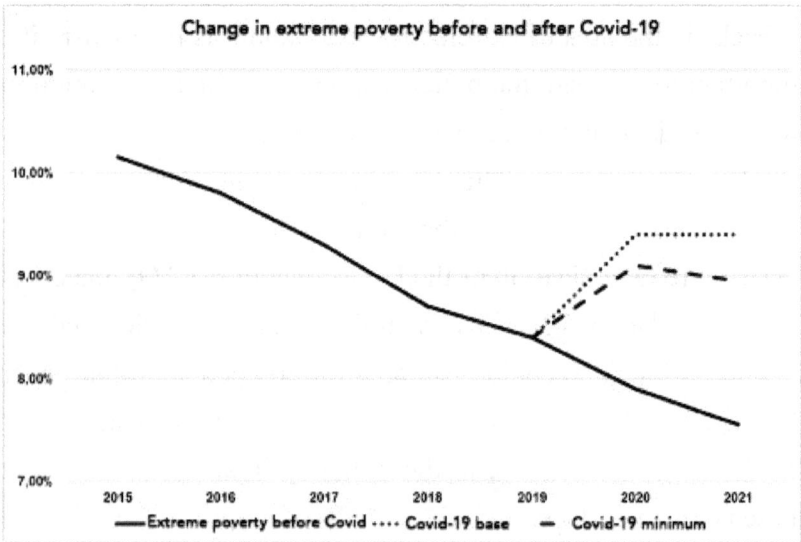

Source: The World Bank Group.

China's experience in defeating extreme poverty, despite

the pandemic and its economic effects, opens another space for study between both parties, especially in the field of cooperation between universities and national and international entities dedicated to defining effective social development policies for Latin America and the Caribbean. All the experience gained as a result of the pandemic, through direct dialogue by Zoom between both sides of the Pacific, may become a good platform for common work in this area.

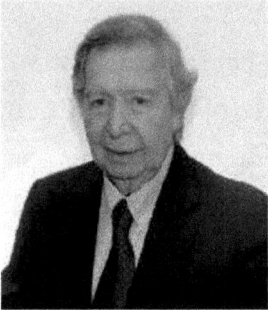

FERNANDO REYES MATTA
(Editor)

Diplomat and Journalist. Director of the Center for Latin American Studies on China, Universidad Andrés Bello, Chile.

Ambassador of Chile to the People's Republic of China, 2006-2010. International Advisor to President Ricardo Lagos, 2000-2006. Ambassador to New Zealand, 1997-2000. Director of Information and Culture, Ministry of Foreign Affairs, 1994-1996.

Media Advisor to the Chile Mission to the United Nations, New York, 1991-1994.

Director, Revista "Diplomacia" (2014-2019), Academia Diplomática de Chile. Coordinator, CELAC-China Project of the Council of International Relations of Latin America (Consejo de Relaciones Internacionals de América Latina, RIAL) (2018/2020). Author of various academic works in collaboration with professional journals and books. Frequent contributing columnist on international affairs. Books: China: Innovación y Tradición. China-América Latina: cómo ir más allá del 2020. Chile-China 40 años: ¿qué trae el futuro? País Pequeño con Mapa Grande, La política exterior de Ricardo Lagos.